YOUR BEST DEFENSE

SMART STRATEGIES
FOR STAYING SAFE

Other books by Wes Manko:

How to be Safe, No Matter What

Color Me Safe: A Woman's Self-Defense Coloring Book

YOUR BEST DEFENSE

SMART STRATEGIES
FOR STAYING SAFE

WES MANKO

HenschelHAUS Publishing, Inc.
Milwaukee, Wisconsin

Published by HenschelHAUS Publishing, Inc.
www.henschelHAUSbooks.com

ISBN: 978159598-480-7
E-ISBN: 978159598-493-7
LCCN: 2017937238

Author photo by Jenny Toutant

Printed in the United States

*This book is dedicated to those who stand up
to the bullies of the world.*

TABLE OF CONTENTS

Author's Note

This book is specifically designed so that you can either read it from start to finish or skip to the chapter(s) most relevant to your individual situation.

DISCLAIMER

The material presented in this book is for educational purposes only. Neither the publisher nor the author makes any representation, warranty, or guarantee that the information or techniques described in this book will be effective in any self-defense situation or otherwise. Neither the author nor the publisher is in any way responsible for injuries that may result from the practice or use of some of the information or techniques presented within. Some self-defense applications may not be justified in some circumstances under applicable federal, state, or local law.

Names used in this book are fictitious to protect people's privacy.

Always check with your local law enforcement agency regarding the use of proper force. Neither the author nor the publisher makes any representation or warranty regarding the legal or ethical appropriateness of any technique mentioned in this book.

Please consult your physician prior to beginning any exercise or physical training program.

FOREWORD

Self-defense expert Wes Manko offers a concise and realistic approach to the problem of violence in our society with this new book. His focus on prevention of violence is a breath of fresh air. This book examines the many possible violent encounters we may face as we go through life and provides ways to avoid and or neutralize them.

While our bones hold the innate rage of centuries of violence, we must also be aware that there are those that wish us harm and how we choose to react will impact our soul. Taking responsibility for personal safety in a manner that doesn't expose us to violence is a good first step.

There is no other book on the market that I am aware of that tackles the issues that every person and every family can face. From learning how to deal with a bully, using knowledge to avoid being a target of rape, making your home and workplace more secure, to dealing with the challenges of terrorism and gun violence, Mr. Manko offers solid and practical wisdom in this book.

His advice comes from the combination of academic achievement in the fields of Police Science and Criminal Justice with many years of teaching self-defense to a diverse clientele of Fortune-500 executives, non-profits, law enforcement, military, and educational institutions. Through this path he has come to understand what the most practical approaches to dealing with violence are without having to engage in physical contact most of the time. He states that self-defense can be like an onion, you have layer upon layer to use before having to engage an attacker physically.

For those of us wishing to yield to the ancient specter of violence in our bones, this is a balm of knowledge can redirect us to being more human while being more safe.

—Resmaa Menakem
author of *My Grandmother's Hands: Racialized Trauma and the Pathway to Mending Our Hearts and Bodies*

CHAPTER ONE
VIOLENCE SURROUNDS US

Violence can strike anywhere and at anytime. It can put us and our loved ones in danger and even cause death. This book is an exploration of how we can better deal with preventing violence—because prevention of violence is our best defense.

HOW IT ALL BEGAN

It was a day that began the same as any other day at the high school. Students scurried to class, teachers taught, and one boy would have his life changed.

The boy, who was emerging into manhood and fancied pursuing an acting career, walked inconspicuously down the hall to his next class. Then without warning, his left shoulder was struck from behind, causing him to spin around and drop his books.

"Hey!" the school bully shouted in the boy's face. "Why'd you hit me?"

Disoriented by the blow and confused, the young man didn't know what to say or how to respond. The school bully had hit him and not vice versa. (Only much later would the boy learn that this is a common technique used by bullies of all ages.)

In about the time it takes to blink, the school bully grabbed the boy by his ankles and lifted him up. The boy felt his head smash into the concrete floor, and his glasses went flying from his face, shattering on the floor, only to be crushed by the bully's large crew. The bully bounced the boy's head against the floor and taunted him in front of a gathered throng of students who had stopped to watch the spectacle.

What seemed like an eternity of pain and torment was over in an instant. As the boy sat crumpled on the hallway floor, one of the bully's gang members handed him back his broken glasses. Spirit-crushing laughter echoed down the hallway, but faces were a mere blur to the boy.

A teacher's voice broke the revelry and ended the torment. "Boys, come with me." It was time to see the school principal.

As the boy trudged along behind the teacher, he anticipated the worst. But he was pleasantly shocked when the principal looked at him, smiled, and said, "Well, I think you learned your lesson." That was it. Somehow, the reaction from the principal was more surprising than the scuffle.

When the boy went to his next class, the gym teacher asked, "Why didn't you kill the guy?" Clearly, the tyrant of the school hallways was despised by the faculty, and more than one teacher would be delighted to see the intimidator beaten. And back in the mid-1970s, what happened in a private school stayed in a private school.

This was a day that shattered many myths for the boy. For almost two years, he had studied a sport martial art and he could have even tested for a brown belt had he not quit to earn some money. *What had gone wrong?*

As he ran the attack scenario over and over in his mind, he realized he had never been trained for this type of attack.

The next class began with another shock. One of the bully's gang members was in his class. The boy pretended not to notice him, but to no avail. He could neither run nor hide.

"Hey, where was your karate today?" the big creep jeered.

Taunting laughter broke out in the classroom. Those who hadn't seen the short-lived fight had certainly heard about it from those who had. With a sick feeling in his stomach, the boy now knew instinctively that the bully would not stop unless he took action. . . immediately.

"After I kick his face in," the boy yelled back, "I'm going to beat the crap out of you!"

The creep, who was bigger than the boy, just smiled and then quickly turned his head the other way without responding. He backed down. The revelation was not missed on the boy, and a plan began to form when he found out that the bully's locker was right outside this classroom.

Finally, the school bell rang, proclaiming the end of the last class of this tortuous day. The boy was determined to at least try to change his misfortune and waited patiently by the bully's locker as the rumor of a new fight spread through the halls like wildfire.

Then the moment of truth came. The boy saw the bully walking toward his locker, but there was something different about him. The thug kept his head down as if to avoid eye contact with the boy.

The boy confronted him. The bully opened his locker but said nothing, so the boy challenged him some more. Finally, when it was clear that the bully was losing whatever respect he might have had from the onlookers, he suddenly threw down his books and charged the boy.

The boy's perfect side kick sent the bully crashing back into the locker, and then something strange happened. The blow did not faze the bully at all. In fact, it just made him angrier. He charged again and this time, the fight ended up on the floor, as most fights do.

In the style of martial art, the boy was learning, there was no ground fighting. Unfortunately for the boy, the bully was a former school wrestler, and the boy quickly found himself beneath the bully. He had to improvise quickly or it would be lights out.

The words of the boy's hero, Bruce Lee, ran through his mind: *Adapt to the fight.* So he started to punch the bully, and even though he was pinned on the ground beneath the bully, he grabbed the bully by the throat with one hand and gained enough leverage to stand up and break free.

Punches flew from left and right. A teacher's voice could be heard shouting from down the hallway, "Stop fighting! Stop fighting!" But those commands weren't even picked up on the radar of the two teen combatants. The boy was getting the worst of the fight, and none of his techniques worked. Suddenly, out of nowhere, the boy shot his fist into the bully's eye. Time froze as the bully flew back several feet. The fight stopped. It was over for the bully. The boy had won.

Although he was pleased to have beaten the bully, the boy was puzzled. His punch was a completely natural movement, and it was not a motion he had been taught in his sport martial arts class. In truth, nothing he had been taught in his two years of classes had been effective in this real fight. *Why?*

The following day, something even stranger happened. The bully's gang, most of whom were taller than the boy, came up to him and apologized for what they had said. Again, he wondered *why*.

The mystery would plague the boy for several years, and ultimately the answer would change his future.

I know, because I was that boy.

Chapter Two
The Importance of Intuition

While the correct attitude plays an important role in conveying the "don't mess with me" message, we must always remember that most crime is an act of opportunity. This applies both to stranger attacks and acquaintance attacks. Even though the correct attitude may remove you from the target list in many cases, there is still the chance that the right opportunity may embolden an attacker to act. This is why we must exercise our intuition.

In his book *The Gift of Fear*, Gavin de Becker states that what intuition means is "to guard, to protect." Intuition by definition is a way that we can protect ourselves. Those feelings we have about something being wrong are generally right. In fact, de Becker puts forth the argument that we can even predict violent behavior.

The use of our intuition allows us to empower two other weapons in our nonviolent defense arsenal, which are awareness and avoidance. According to Chris Thomas and George Dillman, authors of *Humane Pressure Point Self-Defense*,

> Avoiding potential danger is more important than defending yourself if you are attacked—common sense is one of your best weapons. Stay out of circumstances where assaults are common. Be aware of your environment and of areas of

potential danger. Pay attention to who is around you. If a person or a situation makes you feel uncomfortable, leave. Do not worry about being rude or impolite – trust your gut. Often your instinctive awareness of danger will warn you long before your thinking mind can recognize a problem.

While many men feel that intuition is a domain mostly for women, they still recognize that it exists by calling it "gut feeling." So whether you are a man or a woman, you have the same ability to use intuition. Remember, if something feels wrong, it probably is.

Intuition comes to us in many ways. Even dark humor can play a vital role as a life-or-death signal, such as getting a package and making a joke that it might be a bomb. Some victims of bomb attacks made jokes about the mysterious package they got before it blew up and hurt or killed them. Even saying something such as "I'd better open this in the next room before it goes off" is a vital indicator of exactly what might happen.

De Becker lists these messengers of intuition as:

- Nagging feelings
- Persistent thoughts
- Humor
- Wonder
- Anxiety
- Curiosity
- Hunches
- Gut feelings

- Doubt
- Hesitation
- Suspicion
- Apprehension
- Fear

A simple way to identify what intuition is and how it works is to consider that you were born with two voices in your head. One voice is loud, sometimes shrill. It is an "I want it now," ego-type, logical voice. The other voice is a quiet, seldom heard, "do the right thing" voice. The challenge is to listen to the quieter voice of intuition.

For example, let's say you are a single mother waiting in line to buy movie tickets with your six-year-old daughter. A stranger says hello and makes an amusing comment about your daughter. Although he's handsome and charming, he gives you a bad feeling, so you step away from him. After the movie, you stick around and talk with a few friends. One of them offers you a ride to your car, because you parked a fair distance from the theater and it is now dark.

The big voice tells you: "Don't be ridiculous. You don't see that guy anywhere around here, and it would be an imposition on your friend. Plus you would feel really stupid." Nevertheless, the little voice suggests: "Stay with your friend and take the car ride."

You decide to follow the big voice because you don't want to appear foolish. When you take your daughter outside the theater and begin walking to your car, the small voice suggests: "Go back and find your friend and get a ride to your car." But, again, you ignore it. Then, as you walk toward your car, out of the corner of your eye, you think you see something, but the big logical voice says, "It's probably nothing—just your imagination."

As you keep walking, you see your car, but since it is late at night, there are no other cars around it. Now you start to get a funny feeling in your stomach, and you think to yourself that maybe the little voice was right. To assure yourself, you turn around. Out of the shadows, the stranger appears. He's walking right toward you and your daughter. There is no one else around now. He's about thirty feet away and closing in.

Your daughter senses something is wrong and asks, "Mommy, what's wrong?"

"Excuse me, but my car won't start!" the stranger calls out.

At this point, you don't care if you look foolish or not. You grab your daughter, lift her into your arms, and begin to walk faster. As you take another look behind you, the stranger is keeping up.

"Hey, lady. I just want to talk!" he yells.

Your stomach begins to churn as you make a decision to run for it. Your daughter begins to cry. The car is now only a few feet away. You hear heavy footsteps closing in, but you're too scared to look back. You fumble for your keys.

Everything is happening so fast now, but it feels as though you're in slow motion. You have the car key in hand as your reach the car. Quickly you swing open the door and dive in, almost tossing your daughter into the passenger-side seat.

As the lock clicks the car doors shut, the stranger's body slams up against your door. He begins to strike the window with his palms as you start the car engine and floor the pedal. The tires squeal as you pull out of the parking stall.

Why didn't you listen to your intuition? Many of us have found ourselves in a scenario such as this but escaped. For others, the results are tragic.

When we understand how the big voice and little voice work, we can use them to more effectively protect ourselves and our loved ones.

INTUITION DEVELOPMENT EXERCISES

When performing these exercises, try to be as relaxed as possible.

Exercise One

One person stands with his eyes closed while another person tries to sneak up on person #1. The person must identify the direction that the other person is coming from by pointing at him. While this is best suited to be done in a park, any area that is sufficiently large will do.

When doing this exercise indoors, it's good to pick a place where the floor doesn't squeak, as that will give away the direction a person is coming from.

Exercise Two

This is a more challenging variation of Exercise One. This time, three or more people can be involved. One person stays in the middle while the others surround him on four corners, depending on how many players you have. If just three people are involved, then one person stands in the middle between the two others.

With his eyes closed, the person in the middle has to detect who is coming toward him by pointing at them. Only one person should move at a time toward the person in the middle. If the person in the middle points his finger and makes a guess, he can open his eyes to see if he was right. Then the game begins over again. The players can switch places as they wish.

Should the player coming toward the person in the middle not be spotted while the person in the middle still has his eyes closed, the approaching player can tap the person in the middle on the shoulder if he gets close.

Sometimes thinking of walking toward a person will trigger a response.

Exercise Three

This is a far more advanced version of the previous exercise and should only be practiced if the players have done the other two exercises and feel comfortable enough to try this one. It is designed to create more stress while playing this game.

The scenario is the same as with Exercise Two, but this time, players have the option of running to the person in the middle. They can also brush their hand against the throat of the person in the middle if the latter hasn't made a selection in time.

Once the person in the middle points to someone, whether correctly identifying the person or not, the session ends.

Exercise Four

This is a fun game called "Pickpocket." One person puts an piece of paper approximately 6 X 2 inches his belt in the back. Then that person closes his eyes. The other person must snatch the piece of paper that's being held by the belt. The person with the piece of paper in the belt must have his eyes closed and can only stop the other person by sensing him. When he feels that the piece of paper may be snatched away, he can reach for it with his hand and protect it.

This is a great way to develop sensitivity about someone walking in back of you or trying to grab you from behind. Once you practice this enough, you will discover that if the person trying to snatch the paper looks at it long enough, you will be able to sense him and prevent him from getting it.

Exercise Five

This is a group version of the "Pickpocket." There should be at least five or six participants to make this work, but ideally, a group of at least ten works the best. The more people you get for this, the better.

One person is the observer. Everybody else has a 6-by-2-inch piece of paper sticking out of his or her belt in the back and is standing in a circle, which is outlined by a piece of rope on the ground. Parks usually make good areas for this exercise.

While participants have their eyes closed, the observer taps the person who will be the pickpocket. When the observer shouts "Open," everybody in the group begins to walk around with their eyes open.

It is up to the pickpocket to get as many pieces of paper as he can before he gets noticed. Participants can prevent the pickpocket from taking their papers by putting their hand on their back to secure the paper, but they can't keep their hand there all the time—only when they sense the pickpocket is there.

Not only is this a good exercise for developing your sensing ability, but it's fun to play at parties, too. While it may seem strange that having fun is brought up in what should be a serious matter, people learn a lot more quickly when doing enjoyable activities. In addition, you keep practicing those things that are fun. Also, by practicing with a spirit of fun involved, you diminish the stress and fear of an attack.

Exercise Six

Training your peripheral vision is another variation of being able to use your intuition. In this exercise, one person sits in a chair looking straight ahead. The other person comes from behind and starts to move his hand to the top or to either side of the seated person. When the seated person feels the hand coming from behind or sees it in his peripheral vision, he says the direction the hand is coming from, such as right, left, or top.

Exercise Seven

This is an advanced version of the previous exercise. This time, one person stands looking straight ahead while the other person, from behind, uses a long stick, such as the end of a broom handle, to not only move by the three directions past the person's head, but also between the person's legs.

Once the person senses the item and knows the direction it's coming from, he can say left, right, top, or bottom. The idea is to first sense the item, but if that fails, to use peripheral vision to see it. This exercise helps you build up a way to avoid danger before it strikes.

Exercise Eight

Select three swatches of cloth of different colors, say yellow, purple, and green, for example. While you are not looking, have your partner arrange them and cover them with pieces of cardboard. Turn around and try to guess which color is under which piece of cardboard.

CHAPTER THREE

KEEPING YOUR CHILD SAFE

B aby boomers can recall a much safer time in the United States when parents and children could trust anyone. Still, it was a time where some subjects, such as molestation or incest, were not talked about publicly. Molestation, after all, is a nicer word than child sexual assault, which is what it really means.

SELECTING A BABY-SITTER

Most couples do not live close enough to their parents to leave their children in the safe hands of Grandma and Grandpa, and are compelled to go to external resources to obtain childcare.

Unfortunately, the mindset of some parents disregards childcare or babysitting as a real job. For them, it's just a matter of finding the right neighbor's teenager, or if they are more affluent, a professional baby-sitter or nanny. In many cases, more thinking and planning goes into the family vacation than into finding a qualified, trustworthy, mature babysitter.

As a parent, you need to realize that the baby-sitter is an employee into whose care you will entrust your precious children, as well as your possessions, when you hand over the keys to your house. Therefore, doesn't it make sense that you select the most qualified person for the job? Someone you can trust with absolute confidence?

You should be able to garner this level of trust, whether you hire a babysitter or use a home or business daycare provider. Parents sometimes assume that since home or business daycare providers are licensed, they provide safe care. This is not always the case. However, home daycare providers survive by word of mouth and quality of service, which is different than an occasional babysitter who just needs pocket money.

Similarly, business daycare providers can be under scrutiny from co-workers and, in some cases, on-site cameras. That is not to say that problems can't occur in these settings. However, if these services have been around for several years and complaints have not been lodged against them, chances are that they will be safe havens for your children. Nevertheless, be thorough in checking them out first.

As a parent, it is prudent to check any daycare provider's service by:

- Talking to present clients
- Cross-checking the names of employees against a sexual offender registry list
- Checking for any code or criminal violations with the police department or the Better Business Bureau (although most small businesses may not be able to afford membership in that organization).

Use your intuition and incorporate any steps listed below into your examination of home or business daycare providers.

The Three Steps

There are three steps you should use in the babysitter selection process: 1) the application, 2) the interview, and the 3) use of your intuition.

When you receive an inquiry for your babysitting position in response to an ad or from networking with your co-workers and friends, you can do a brief interview over the phone if it's someone you don't know. Keep the questions simple, such as the person's availability, prior experience, and age. This gives you a chance to use your intuition to see how the applicant "feels." If she passes the initial test, then get the person's address and send out an application. I use the word "she" in reference to the babysitter because most babysitters are female. It is also important to note that, statistically, males are far more likely than females to assault a child.

1. The Application

Once you've conducted a favorable telephone interview, ask for the person's address for where to send the application. The application form should include writing space for the applicant's name, address, phone number, and the names of references, as well as their addresses and phone numbers. Other vital information you should require: past dates of service, whom to contact in case of emergency, and whether or not the applicant knows child CPR or has had any medical training that deals with saving children's lives.

When you receive the application, you can judge the seriousness of the applicant by how comprehensively the questions are answered, as well as by how the form looks.

From there, you can select candidates for the next step in the process.

2. The Interview

Once you have selected the candidates you want to interview, call the people who are listed as references on the application and talk to them. Ask open-ended questions, such as "What is Linda like?" and "How long has she been babysitting? Do you know others who have used her as a babysitter? And How do you know her?" Also, ask references if they know anyone else you can talk to about the applicant. Once you get those names, call the other referrals up and talk to them.

Questions such as "Does Linda hang around any bad people?" may not get you straight answers, as opposed to open-ended questions, such as "Tell me about her friends" and "What do she and her friends like to do?"

Another good question might be, "How old is her boyfriend?" This question assumes she has a boyfriend, and the reference person is more likely to open up to you. Also, if she doesn't have a boyfriend, you will get straight answers. If she does have a boyfriend, ask for his age. If Linda is 16 and her boyfriend is 30, you might have a problem. Your antennae should go up, depending on the answers you receive.

Using this interview strategy sends a message to the applicant that you are thorough. There may be some applicants who will be discouraged by your questions, but this is a good thing. You want what is best for your child and yourself, so don't worry about hurting the applicant's feeling. On the bright side, this painstaking process will help you worry less when you are away.

After calling all the references, move on to selecting the most promising candidates for a face-to-face interview. While this can be mostly a cerebral process, try to keep in touch with your feelings. A bad feeling can mean a bad choice.

After evaluating the feedback from the references, ask yourself whether or not you could trust this person with your child. What intuitive feeling do you get when you ask this?

3. The Questions

When asking questions of the applicant, watch her reactions. How she reacts will give you a good or bad feeling. Listen to your intuition and write down your answers. Perhaps even have a form to fill out for each candidate so that you can review later.

Here are some key questions you should ask:

◆ "How do you discipline children?"
◆ "What discipline methods did your parents use?"
◆ "Did your parents ever use physical punishment?"

Babysitters who were physically abused as children may have a greater predilection to physically punish as well. Moreover, she may use the same method that was used on her.

- "In your experience, have you ever come across a child who was physically abused or sexually molested? If yes, what did you do about it? Did you report it to the police?"

- "What do you like about this work?"

- "Have you taken care of younger siblings?"

- "What don't you like about this line of work?"

- "Describe the best babysitting experience you have ever had."

- "Describe the worst babysitting experience you have ever had."

- "What would you do if the lights in the house go out?"

- "What would you do if the child gets sick?"

- "What would you do if the child stopped breathing?"

- "What would you do if the child began to choke?"

- "Tell me about a problem in your life and how you solved it."

- "Tell me about a problem in your life and how someone helped you with it."

- "What do you think of drugs and alcohol?"

- "Do you have a best friend? Tell me about your relationship with him or her."

- "What would you do if a child played with herself/himself or did an inappropriate act?"

- "What would you do if a child asked you to keep a secret from the parents?"

- "How do you break up fights between siblings?"

- "Can we test you for drugs?"

- "Do you personally know anyone you would not allow around our child or children in general? Who is this person?"

- "Do you have a boyfriend? What is your relationship with him? Will he be visiting you when you are baby-sitting?"

These questions probe for maturity and responsibility. If an applicant talks little about her good experiences and a lot about her bad ones, that is a clue. Also, if she uses negative terms such as "brat" to describe her experience with a child, you should dismiss her as a candidate.

If at anytime you feel you are not getting a complete answer, feel free to use the silent treatment. Don't say anything unless you hear more from the applicant.

Finally, encourage the applicant to ask you any questions. Specifically, she should be asking questions that explore what your rules are, if the children have any medical conditions, what activities you recommend for the children to do, and what television programs the children should or should not watch. All such inquiries demonstrate a good deal of responsibility. If the applicant does not ask these types of questions, you need to beware that perhaps the candidate is not appropriate to watch your children.

THE RULES
Once you have settled on a candidate, it is time to discuss the rules, such as:

- Don't take the kids out of the house.

- Don't bathe the kids.

Establish your rules, write them down and post them in a visible place (like the refrigerator), make them crystal clear, and never allow them to be changed. Be sure your children are also aware of these rules and have them contact you if these rules are not obeyed. In an emergency, they can use a code word. Of course, this depends on the ages of the children.

Circuit Breakers, Emergency Protocols

After you have reviewed expectations, show the babysitter the circuit breaker panel and teach her how to fix the breakers if they go off. If your house has a fuse box, show her how to change burned-out fuses. Show her the fire extinguisher, and make sure she knows how to operate it. Tell her about the smoke alarm protocols. Show her the child's medical release form and give her relevant contact numbers in case of an emergency. Post a similar list on the refrigerator or easily accessible location.

You're on Candid Camera

Purchase a camera or cameras that can be hidden and set it up. Not only will this give you added peace of mind, recorded images can be valuable source of evidence if your child is somehow hurt or harmed.

Additional Reading

One of the best and most comprehensive books on the subject of keeping children and teenagers safe is called *Protecting the Gift* by former FBI profiler Gavin de Becker. This book highly insightful and easy to read; I highly recommend that you read it.

PUBLIC PLACES

In every parent's life, there comes a time when the child must venture into the public. The key is to have the child prepared well enough to deal with whatever negative situations might come along. Here are some "Best Defense" tips:

♦ Because anyone can buy a badge and give the appearance of being a policeman or security person, tell your child to seek out a woman if they become lost. Statistically, a woman is less likely to harm them than a man.

♦ When you tell a child that certain men will harm them, they picture an unshaven bum and not a man in a suit or nicer clothing. That's a problem.

♦ Remember, for every person in public places who might hurt your child, there are thousands who won't.

♦ A child who is trained to approach strangers correctly is less likely to become a victim than a child who is taught to never talk to strangers.

♦ To train your child to talk to strangers, ask your child to pick out a stranger, approach the unknown person, ask that person for the time of day or for directions to a particular place. Afterward, ask your child why s/he chose that particular person, if he/she felt comfortable with that person, and if s/he had a sense that the person felt comfortable with them.

♦ Teach your children that certain situations can make seemingly safe locations dangerous. If a child is told that the mall is a dangerous place, but s/he spends lots of time there without feeling threatened, s/he will disregard your message.

However, if you describe the situations at the mall that open the door to danger, such as talking with a man who offers her/him something for free, you help focus your child's attention on specifics that won't be forgotten.

♦ Dress your children in highly visible clothing that will allow you to spot them in a crowd.

♦ Before you go into a public place, agree on a specific place to meet if you get separated.

♦ Use GPS trackers on the children's smartphones

WHAT YOUR CHILDREN SHOULD KNOW BEFORE THEY GO OUT

♦ Teach your children their address and phone number.

♦ Tell your children that if a man, any man, starts to talk to them or come close to them, they should run to a safe place and/or yell for help. They should not talk to or respond to men, regardless of how harmless they appear or if they claim to need some type of help.

♦ Tell your kids to always stay a good distance from any man, and if for some reason they are grabbed, they should yell "He's not my daddy" and fight back.

♦ The best way youngsters can fight back is to do so naturally—bite, scratch, punch, and kick—which they already know how to do without training. Children may not remember choreographed movements or memorized techniques when they are afraid. Children just need a parent's okay to fight back.

♦ Define a *stranger* to a child as anyone whom the child does not know and/or someone your child gets a bad feeling about. Sometimes your child might get a bad feeling from a relative or a known person in a position of authority. Your child should know that every time he or she gets a bad feeling about someone, regardless of who the person is, your child should tell you.

♦ A male stranger may pretend that his is the father of a child the child knows. He'll say he'll call his child on a cell phone and have the other kid talk to yours, but this is just a trick to get the child into his hands as soon as the child comes close to the cell phone.

♦ It's okay to get away from anyone who makes them feel uncomfortable.

♦ Ensure your children that they can always tell you anything, regardless of how bad it is.

♦ It's okay to say "no" to adults.

♦ It's okay to not do what adults tell them if they're alone and if what's being asked will harm or hurt them

♦ Tell them to go to a woman to ask for help.

♦ Teach your kids how to say what's wrong.

♦ It's okay to scream and yell if they are in trouble.

♦ It's okay to run from people who want to harm them.

♦ It's okay to scratch, bite, hit, and kick anyone who is hurting them and/or if someone is touching them in places they don't want to be touched.

♦ It's okay to yell, "This is not my father!" when a man tries to grab them or is holding them against their will.

♦ It's okay to yell even if someone tells them not to yell.

♦ It's okay and safe to tell you when someone tells them to not tell you something. Make sure they do tell. When someone says that something is a secret, your child should always tell you.

♦ Teach your children not to believe someone who says, "Do as you're told, or I'll hurt you." This is a scare tactic.

This is not to say children who are kidnapped are not hurt or even killed, but if the criminal is going to do this anyway, there is no down side for the child to resist.

◆ Have a safe word known only to your children and people they can trust to pick them up from school.

◆ Ensure that your children never leave an area with someone they don't know, even if that someone is ordering them to go.

◆ When children are old enough to walk to transportation or to/from school, they should have a cell phone with emergency numbers programmed in.

◆ If your children are going to walk to school, go with them and study every possible route. If you get a bad feeling from a particular route, tell your children not to follow it.

Also, if your children are small for their age, they should go in a group. You and the other parents should know the names and contact information for all group members.

Never allow very small children to walk to school alone. The criterion for being too small to go out alone is this: if the father can pick the child up and easily tuck him/her under his arm and the child cannot escape from his grip.

◆ Develop your children's intuition by pointing to strangers and asking your kids if they would trust that stranger to help them. If not, why not? You can even turn this into a game for the child.

◆ If your children are old enough or mature enough for cell phones, get them one. Program the cell phone so that hitting one number can speed-dial 911, and train the child to use it.

Even if children are kidnapped or abducted, they may be able to reach into their pocket and hit that button. There are also apps that can track cell phones.

AT HOME

Many parents are concerned about determining the appropriate age when a child may be left at home alone. The main concern should not necessarily be the child's age, but rather maturity and necessity. Ideally, a child should never be left alone, but because of unforeseen circumstances, it can happen. Consequently, here are some actions parents can take:

♦ If a child is left all alone at home, the child should never respond to a knock on the door or answer the door, regardless of who is outside.

Even if there is an adult in the house, the child should not answer the door. Children may be too small to see through a peephole to verify a person's identity. Criminals are good at giving convincing reasons to enter a home. Some may even dress up as authority figures and carry badges.

♦ Children left at home should have the ability to contact their parents as quickly as possible, as well as know the emergency numbers for the police and fire departments.

♦ Should a fire or other dangerous situation occur in the home, children should have a safe place in the neighborhood to which they can run.

♦ While nothing has a 100 percent guarantee, the more precautions a parent takes, the safer the child becomes.

BULLIES

When Sally found out her son was being bullied at school, she enrolled him in a martial arts class so he could learn to defend himself. She felt that if she intervened in some way, he would be far worse off. Her son, Brad, learned quickly in his class and felt confident that he could fight the bully if it became necessary.

The chance soon arose. When the bully began to intimidate and push Brad around, Brad did exactly as he'd been taught and executed a perfect takedown, causing the bully to smack the concrete. But no sooner had he dropped the bully than the bully's ten-plus gang members tore into Brad, ultimately hospitalizing him.

While hoping to instill confidence in her son, Sally made two mistakes. The first was not getting the school authorities involved. The second was having her son learn from someone who was more oriented in teaching a sport martial art rather than reality-based martial art.

Preventing violence in school requires a multi-faceted approach. It involves getting the school officials involved. Many schools now have security guards who can keep an eye out for trouble, but they need to know what trouble may occur. Parents should use all the tools at their disposal to keep their children safe, even if it means getting the police, teachers, and other parents involved.

Having children learn proper self-defense provides the parent with the peace of mind that their offspring have a back-up plan, whether they are in or out of school. However, parents also need to know what works and what doesn't. For instance, most of today's martial arts teaches students to only deal with one attacker at a time. This simply doesn't work in the real world, where a person may face multiple assailants at the same time, especially in a public setting such as a school.

One reality-based martial art that has a proven track record of dealing with multiple attackers is a Russian martial art called *Systema*, "The System," which is currently being used by the Russian special forces because of its effectiveness. It is also being taught to some military and law enforcement personnel in the United States and worldwide.

Other considerations in selecting the proper type of martial art include the practicality of the teaching. How long do students have to wait before being is taught something practical.

How can a parent distinguish between a sport and a self-defense martial art? In today's world, it is hard to tell one from another, as many martial artists advertise that what they teach is self-defense. Some teachers who teach a sport martial art do tell their students what works as a self-defense and what doesn't, while others don't.

Here are a few clues that will allow you to determine if a martial art is a sport, rather than being reality-based. Sport martial arts instructors generally will:

- Participate in tournaments.
- Teach mostly one-on-one defenses rather than defenses against group attacks.
- Be focused mostly on cardiovascular development, fitness, and discipline rather than on going self-defense

that includes defenses from standing, sitting and ground work.

◆ Do a lot of practice on striking pads instead of striking each other. With proper instruction, one can learn how to absorb blows without being injured.

◆ Select people of the same height, weight, and skill level to practice with each other. Attackers come in various sizes and weights.

◆ Not teach how to avoid physical confrontations without using force.

◆ Not teach methods that allow a smaller individual to bring down a larger one, but instead focus on pairing students of same height and weight.

◆ Not teach defenses against group attacks.

◆ Not teach defense against grabs, locks, chokes and group attacks both from an individual and a group scenario.

◆ Not teach defenses against knives and guns.

◆ Not teach proper use of body mechanics, breathing, tensing and relaxing.

◆ Not teach proper use of breathing for blow absorption.

◆ Not teach situational awareness nor intuition development.

There are, however, exceptions to the rules. The following do teach self-defense techniques: boxing, Thai kick-boxing, mixed martial arts (MMA), Krav Maga (Israeli self-defense training), and some forms of jujitsu, to name a few. This is important for parents to know, because if they are told by a martial arts instructor that classes teach students how to deal with group attacks, parents need to find out if the instructor means that the person being attacked is defending against one person at a time or a group. Bullies and their crews aren't going to be polite and follow rules. They will attack at the same time, and there are no rules.

Of course, bullying can happen to girls, too. Jennifer was twelve when another girl in her art class threatened to beat her up. Frightened and not knowing what to do, she asked her father for help that evening. Fortunately, her father had a background in dealing with issues such as this. He told her to challenge the girl to a one-on-one match after school, and to challenge her in front of her gang. The wording she was supposed to use was very specific. She was to tell the girl: "Just me and you out back after school."

Needless to say, Jennifer was very frightened. She tried to believe her father was right, but that didn't stop the upset feeling she had.

When the next art class began, the bully and her gang started in on Jennifer, who reached down deep inside herself and made the challenge. The bully quickly agreed. When the school bell rang, Jennifer started to become more frightened. She made her way down the long corridor, out the door, and into the schoolyard where she was supposed to fight.

No one was there, so she waited. Ten minutes passed and still no bully. She began to become more confident. Another ten minutes passed and still no bully. Finally, after waiting half an hour, she started to walk home. At the next art class, the bully and her crew showed up, but this time, they didn't pick on Jennifer or anyone else in the class.

In this case, as opposed to Sally's story, Jennifer's father was qualified to come up with the appropriate response, which had nothing to do with learning a physical defense tactic.

Rather, it involved the use of psychology. Effective self-defense involves not only physical movements, but also awareness, intuition, correct breathing, proper body mechanics, relaxation, as well as psychology. It is always best to prevent a fight rather than have to take part in one, regardless of how much self-defense training one has had.

Still, there are a number of concerns any parent would have about Jennifer's situation, despite this happy ending. Weapons, especially firearms, are finding their way more easily into the classroom. In Jennifer's case, the bully didn't have a record of using knives or guns. In fact, her ability to manipulate people just came from the fear of an attack rather than actual violence, and Jennifer's father knew that.

But what if the other girl had a knife and was willing to use it? Would the story be different if the bully lived in the neighborhood? What would have happened if the school authorities had been involved?

While this instance ended peacefully, each incident is different, and there is no formula for guaranteed solutions.

As schoolchildren mature, for the most part, they want to take things on by themselves. Therefore, having good communication between parent and child is essential. While this scenario did not involve school authorities, it is always advisable that the school counselor or other proper authorities know a child is a bully or being bullied. Unfortunately, the bottom line is that some children will take matters into their own hands.

Bullies usually target students who are loners, appear weak, or don't seem to fit in, because one of the last things a bully wants to deal with is someone who has a crew of friends. Therefore, if students join a club or clubs, they increase their chances of not being picked on, especially if they are always walking around with a group of friends. If a student becomes a target of a bully, the friends only need put their hands on victim's shoulders and just walk the student away from the bully without saying a word. This will leave the bully target-less.

Even in the most elite of schools, students know where they can hide from school cameras. Bullies will take advantage of this.

In addition, part of effective anti-bullying training involves learning how to fall and absorb strikes without getting injured.

If a bully lives in the neighborhood, children should feel open and safe about discussing any bullying incident with their parents. Then the parents can contact the parents of the bully to resolve the issue. If this doesn't work, the police should be called. While some police might not wish to get involved in a bullying scenario, when the terminology used to explain the incident to the authorities contains such catch phrases as, "attempted assault," "assault," or "attempted murder," their resolve to assist increases.

Signs of Bullying

In his book, *So I Won't Have to Fight: Bully Solutions From Martial Arts Masters,* author Brad Scornavacco identifies what parents can look for as warning signs to determine if their the child is being bullied. These include physical signs, behavioral signs, and emotional signs. According to Scornavacco:

"Physical signs of bullying include.

- ◆ Torn or damaged clothing, books (ruined in an attack)

- ◆ Missing possessions (stolen or destroyed)

- ◆ Cuts, bruises or scratches the child doesn't want to talk about or gives parents lame excuses, especially recurring injuries

Behavioral signs of bullying include:

- ◆ Has few if any friends with whom he or she spends time

- ◆ Is afraid of going to school, riding the school bus or taking part in organized activities with peers (such as clubs)

- ◆ Changes his or her route when walking to and from school with no reason

- ◆ Has lost motivation to do school work. Grades may drop and assignments may not be getting turned in

Emotional signs of bullying are:

- ◆ Appears sad, moody, teary or depressed after school

- ◆ Can't sleep or has recurring bad dreams

- ◆ Often has headaches stomachaches or other physical pain

♦ Has little or no appetite or develops strange eating habits

♦ Appears anxious and suffers from low self-esteem."

Cyber-Bullying

This is a form of bullying that can reach children or teenagers where they now live—which is social media. Unlike physical bullying, there are no bruises. However, this form of bullying can be just as deadly, if not more so, as a number of those bullied young people have committed suicide.

The best responses to cyber-bullying is having a good self-image and effective communication between the child's parents and/or teachers. Parents should discuss this subject with their children at an early age and develop a plan to deal with it. A rule of thumb is to have this conversation before the child is plugged into social media. Parents can limit or set rules for technology use, but kids being kids, they can and do get around such limitations.

The key is ensuring that the child knows that he or she has control over emotions in response to a cyber-bullying attack.

The good thing about social media is that children can "block" their attackers. Other strategies that have been employed are to ignore the attacker or use humor against the attacker. If attackers know they are not getting what they want, they will move on.

This does not mean that the attack should not get reported. That is a choice between the one being bullied and his/her parents. The most important thing to remember is that when good communication exists between parent and child to the extent that the child feel comfortable telling parents everything, then there is a less likelihood that cyber-bullying will be effective.

It is equally important for parents to ask bullied children about their energy level after the event. If they say their energy level is higher or there is no change, then they are okay. If they say their energy level is low, it is possible that thoughts of suicide are present.

CHAPTER FOUR
KEEPING TEENAGERS SAFE

There are many dangers facing teenagers these days. In his book *Protecting the Gift*, Gavin de Becker states that "gunshot wounds are now the leading cause of death for boys in America." This statement, while horrific, illustrates the change in times, attitudes, and easy access to guns from the 1950s to the present.

For parents, the concept of bullying they most likely relate to is one that dates back to the time when they were in school. This may mean that they see bullying as a one-on-one issue with participants being of close to equal weight and without any other considerations. For the most part, this notion is pretty close to fiction. As we discussed in the previous chapter, teenagers can be bullied by people twice their size, and some have guns and are in gangs.

The best weapon a parent has under these circumstances is an open line of communication with their child. If your child wants to talk to you, put everything else on the sidelines, including work. Opt for adopting a *life* ethic rather than a *work* ethic. Transferring work to the back burner is very hard to do in American society, especially when both parents work and may often involve extremely long hours. This can lead to miscommunications and feelings by children that their parents don't care about them. Some teenagers won't demand your time because they are trying to prove to themselves that they can handle any situation. But this attitude, if taken to the extreme, can lead to school massacres.

So how can you tell if your teenager is prone to commit these types of acts? In *Protecting the Gift*, author Gavin de Becker notes predictive signals that occur prior to major acts of violence. They are:

- Alcohol and drug abuse
- Addiction to media products, pornography
- A sense of aimlessness
- A fascination with weapons and violence
- Experience with guns
- Access to guns
- Sullen, angry, depressed (SAD)
- Seeking status and worth through violence
- Threats of violence or suicide
- Rejection and humiliation
- Media provocation

THE POTENTIAL FOR VIOLENCE

Bullies act out learned aggression, which usually stems from their life experiences. This could mean being exposed to domestic violence and believing that such behavior is normal. The old adage that the apple doesn't fall far from the tree surely applies here.

If we know what can cause this violence, how do we prevent it? More specifically, if your family doesn't have these problems, what can you do to ensure that the product of such dysfunctional problems doesn't impact your teenager at school?

Besides having open lines of communication between parent and child, students must also be able to identify the signals of potential danger and tell parents and school authorities.

Every school should have psychologist or counselors on hand to deal with this danger.

Many students internalize stress from home, as well as from school, and need a healthy outlet where they can bond beyond their cliques. Parents should encourage and support their teens in accessing these outlets.

Overworked parents and overstressed kids are a combined recipe for disaster. Ideally, corporations should follow the European model and give employees at least four weeks of vacation each year. The key for parents is ensuring that they find time for their children, and to stop what they're doing and really be there. No matter how busy a day is, parents should find time to spend with their children over the dinner table, even if it's just for dessert. Focus on your children's needs, and you'll get a clear picture of what's in their hearts.

The biggest villain in the world today is stress. The more ways you and your family can reduce it, the better. This may mean cutting down on some sport activity or a work project just to spend a weekend together as a family. Slowing down can help people live better. Family mediation practice can help relieve stress and encourage family members to be more open with one another.

Teen Suicide

Teenagers often turn inward when feeling rejected or unwanted. Consequently, they may end up believing that their only form of release is suicide. The American Academy of Child and Adolescent Psychiatry provides this list of symptoms that may occur before deadly suicide attempt:

- Change in eating and sleeping habits.

- Saying things such as "I won't be a problem much longer," "It's no use," or "Nothing matters"

- A marked personality change.

- Drug and alcohol use.

- Rebellious behavior, running away, or violent actions.

- Ongoing boredom, difficulty in concentrating, or a decline in the quality of work.

- Loss of interest in pleasurable activities.

- Frequent complaints about physical symptoms related to emotions, such as headaches and fatigue.

- Putting their affairs in order, such as giving away their favorite possessions, cleaning their room, and throwing away important belongings.

When parents notice such indications in their child or even someone else's child, they should seek professional help as soon as they can. Ensure teens that it's important for them to tell their parents or other authority figure if they see these symptoms in one of their schoolmates—it could mean difference between life and death.

CHAPTER FIVE
WHAT TO TEACH YOUR DAUGHTER ABOUT DATING

In the discussion of violence, we are talking about combat conditioning. While gender conditioning has often been used as an excuse as to why women may be more reluctant to fight back, the fact is that human beings grow up not wanting to hurt other human beings. Violence and hurting others must be taught and conditioned.

Overcoming the fear of getting hurt is just as important as overcoming the fear of hitting someone. That is why it is important to do proper breathing and stress reduction to avoid injury when getting hit and to psychologically accept getting hit and hitting others. ial Art curriculum involves these tactics.

In many of my seminars, I ask women to raise their hands if they would use a particularly horrific physical technique to defend themselves—one that would truly hurt an assailant. About 98 percent of the women reply that they would not, even if it meant losing their own life. Then I ask them if they would use that same technique if they were forced to protect their child. One hundred percent of the women say that they would.

Keep in mind that when you are looking for self-defense training for children who are five years old or younger, the best defense is just letting them know that it is okay to scratch, punch, kick, bite, and scream at any adult who intends to harm them, touch them in an inappropriate place, or move them to another location.

Family self-defense workshops provide a valuable opportunity to have defensive tactics individualized for each participant's physical abilities. In many classes, a person's height or ability to move are not considered. Such self-defense classes are ideal at any age.

Woman's self-defense workshops are also an option if your daughter is ready to start dating or is going off to college. The focus of these workshops should include using psychology to avoid an attack, getting information about where most rapes happen on campus, learning physical escape tactics, practical and natural self-defense techniques against single and multiple attackers, what to do if she encounters a date-rape drug and how to deal with the stress of physical combat in order to avoid injury.

Prior to actually dating, boys and girls may tend to experiment with each other. Older parents can recall the term "playing house." If this concerns you as a parent— and it should—two things can help: open and honest communication and constant vigilance.

Nothing is a 100-percent solution, but if you tell your daughter that it's healthy to be curious and that she should come to you if she has any questions, this may help alleviate some of the concern.

Don't just hold your breath and hope that nothing bad happens. Take an active role, talk to your kids, and give them the information and understanding they need.

If you give them a healthy, age-appropriate perspective on sex, you eliminate much of the mystery about sex, as well as the reasons so many kids get into trouble, especially with social media being so prevalent.

While preparing your daughter for the dating scene should be more than a laundry list chat, it often isn't. It is your responsibility to instruct your daughter on the seriousness of dating and of the qualities she should be looking for in a young man. No one can influence her more than you can as a parent. Hopefully, the wisdom you impart to her will keep her safe from situations with men that require her to act in self-defense. But it is irresponsible to not prepare her for the possibility.

Here are some key concepts every young woman needs to know:

♦ No one has the right to force you to do something you don't want to do or don't want them to do to you.

♦ When you find yourself alone with a guy and you want him to leave, use commands such as "Stop!" or "No!" or "Get out!" If this doesn't work, swear at him with a command. If that doesn't work, excuse yourself to go to the bathroom, lock the door and call for help.

♦ It's best to raise your voice when using commands, although you should not be yelling.

♦ Don't smile when you say "no," because some men won't take you seriously. While this is the man's fault, your response must be effective.

♦ Always have a cell phone with you and set the speed dial to 911, depending on location.

- Tell your parents if something bad happened on the date.

- Always tell the truth.

- Know it's okay to hit, bite, scratch, kick, punch, and gouge your date if he is not listening to you, not respecting you, or doing what you don't want him to do.

- Know that some men will try to slip date rape drugs into your drink to render you defenseless. These drugs may also be put into ice cubes, so be wary of whom you trust at a party.

- Keep your drink with you at all times, even if you have to use the bathroom.

- It's always good to go to a party with female friends who won't desert you. Agree together that even if one of you meets a cute boy, you won't leave with him alone that night.

- When you go on vacation, whether in a place your familiar with or in a foreign place, make sure that in the evening, you never get separated from your female friends or family members, and that all of you return to your hotel together.

Give your daughter emergency money to use if she gets into trouble, and tell her that you love her very much. There is nothing more powerful than giving your daughter the sense that you love her unconditionally.

CHAPTER SIX
PREVENTING COLLEGE RAPE

Depending on the source, statistics indicate that one in five or one in four women will be sexually assaulted on campus. One wonders why self-defense classes are not overflowing with students. The reason is that there is a misconception about self-defense classes.

Some woman may have had experience with sport martial arts. They likely came to the realization that it would take too long to become proficient or felt that they needed to be athletes to protect themselves.

The reality is that there is a difference between sport martial arts and self-defense, or as it is often referred to, reality-based martial arts. Practical self-defense training goes beyond just physical applications. It is layered to encompass prevention and verbal and psychological tactics.

MANY ATTACKERS ARE KNOWN
According to the Rape, Abuse, & Incest National Network (R.A.I.N.N.), every 107 seconds, an American is sexually assaulted. Approximately 2/3 of assaults are committed by someone known to the victim, with 38 percent of the rapists being friends or acquaintances and 44 percent of the victims are under 18, while 80 percent are under the age of

30. An incredible 68 percent of sexual assaults are not reported to the police and 98 percent of rapists will never spend a night in jail. (As with all statistics, these are already outdated once they appear in print. Please refer to the www.rainn.org website for the latest figures.)

The use of alcohol and drugs pose a significant danger. "Various drugs are used to facilitate rape. Alcohol is by far the most frequently used. In a national study of college students, 75 percent of males and 55 percent of females involved in date rape had been drinking or using drugs prior to the assault. Alcohol impairs inhibitions, judgment and decision-making," reports the University Health Services at Berkley. Warning signs of being drugged include:

♦ Feeling drunk when you haven't had a lot of alcohol
♦ Difficulty breathing
♦ Nausea
♦ A sudden increase in feeling dizzy, disoriented or experiencing blurred vision
♦ A body temperature change that can be signaled by chattering teeth or sweating
♦ Finally, waking up with no memory or missing large amounts of memories.

Also keep in mind that a person may pass out before experiencing the full level of these symptoms, depending on what drug is used and in what dosage.

Alcohol is a tool often used by rapists. In some cases, they will use an "overproof," a drink that has more than the normal 40 percent alcohol content. *Everclear* is a type of alcohol that is 151 proof, or more than 50 percent. A potential rapist will slip an overproof alcohol into a woman's drink to get her as drunk as quickly as possible.

According to an article published in 2006 by the Society for the Study of Social Problems by Elizabeth Armstrong, Laura Hamilton, and Brian Sweeney, entitled "Sexual Assault on Campus: A Multilevel, Integrative Approach to Party Rape,"

> The tight link between alcohol and sexual assault suggests that many sexual assaults that occur on college campuses are 'party rapes.'

A recent report by the U.S. Department of Justice defines "party rape" as a distinct form of rape, one that "occurs at an off-campus house or on- or off-campus fraternity and involves . . . plying a woman with alcohol or targeting an intoxicated woman."

While party rape is classified as a form of acquaintance rape, it is not uncommon for the woman to have had no prior interaction with the assailant.

An article by blogger and feminist Jessica Valenti in *The Guardian* found that "numerous studies have found that men who join fraternities are three times more likely to rape, that women in sororities are 74 percent more likely to experience rape than other college women, and that one in five women will be sexually assaulted in the four years away at school." The article concluded that frat brothers rape 300 percent more often than standard male students.

While efforts are underway to curtail these attacks, there are tactics that can be employed to minimize and or eliminate the chances of being assaulted:

- Find out where on campus most sexual assaults have occurred from the Campus Police. If there is a location or frat house that has a bad reputation, stay away from it.

- Take a self-defense course from a qualified, reality-based, instructor. To be most effective, the course should help remove the psychological barrier that human beings have which prevents them from striking someone. It should also remove the fear of getting hit because in a fight, you will get hit. How your body process that strike will impact on your ability to defend yourself.

  Don't choose a course just because it is on campus. Research the instructor's background. Then decide. It is good to have an instructor who not only has expertise in self-defense, but has additional qualifications, such as academic degrees in Criminal Justice or Police Science, has a law enforcement background, or is published on the topic. A good class should also include verbal and psychological tactics, as well as the physical ones.

- Go to events with friends and use a code word to let them know you need help to leave. It could be as simple as "Did you see my red purse?"

- Lie if you have to. Deception is part of effective self-defense.

- If someone has grabbed you and is dragging you off to the bathroom or to a private area, yell for help and if you can, bite his hand. If there are a lot of people at a party, fall down and yell for help. Create a scene if you have to.

♦ Create a good Samaritan policy on campus , if there isn't one already. This states that if someone is calling for help and a person seeing or hearing that person does not respond, they could be fined or expelled.

♦ Bring a tactical flashlight (one with over 120 lumens and a strobe function) that can be employed to temporarily distract an attacker before you are grabbed. The effectiveness of this depends on the amount of light in the location. The bezel of most tactical flashlights has a jagged edge that can be used to strike. If you have a multiple-function flashlight and want to use it for self-defense, keep it on strobe mode all the time.

♦ If possible, bring a rubber door stop in case you need to barricade yourself from an intruder. The door stop can be obtained from any hardware store and if placed on the ground next to a door, you can used it to stop the door from opening toward you. There are also electronic doorstops that incorporate an alarm.

♦ Tell your friends who are not going to the party you are, where you will be and when to phone you to check on you.

♦ Agree on a specific time to leave the event and stick to it.

♦ Bring a cell phone with you and have it set to the person or agency you wish to contact first.

♦ Bring enough money or a credit card in case you need to use a cab.

DATING IN COLLEGE

Evidence shows that most women are attacked by someone they know. This makes dating a top safety concern.

Today's tech world means it's easier to run a background check, although keep in mind, juvenile records are sealed, so only crimes committed beginning at age eighteen will be listed. Before going on a date with someone, go to your state's courthouse website and enter the person's name. Some places may ask or require a birthdate. In Wisconsin, this is called CCAP or Wisconsin Circuit Court Access. Other court data like marriages and divorces will be listed there as well.

An ideal meeting place for a first date is a location where alcohol is not served, such as a coffee shop. Always have your own transportation available rather then be picked up by your date. Pay attention to your intuition. If you're getting a funny feeling about your date, cancel or reschedule the get-together. If the feeling comes again, pay attention to it. If you get a feeling about not going to an event, don't go.

When you have a situation where you bring the man over to your location and he won't leave, you have a number of options. While it is customary to be polite and ask him to leave, some men are wired to ignore this and try to overcome your objections. Therefore, if you give an excuse such as having homework to do, his response may be that you are so intelligent that you don't need to do it tonight.

This can go on and on until the male whittles down your resistance to his advances. Think of the male as a dog. This is not to disparage males, but to provide a visual in terms of how males respond to certain instructive stimuli, such as commands.

To apply the commanding voice technique, raise your voice just below a shout and issue a command, such as

"Please leave now" or "Go home now," or "I want you to leave right now." Most men will gain some sense as to what they are doing and leave.

Some men will ask, "Oh, you'd like me to go?" The answer should be a firm "yes." On the other hand, some men will not leave. If this is the case, drop some swear words with your loud command. One of the most likely reactions you'll receive is, "Oh, you want me to go?"

Men who were raised by parents in an environment where they could get away with anything they wanted until one of the parents used a curse word have, in some cases, become conditioned to keep doing what they are doing until they hear one.

At that point, most of the problem should have been solved. If it has not, then the situation could get dangerous very quickly.

Change your tactic to saying you need to use the restroom. Most men will understand this. Excuse yourself and go to the bathroom. A cell phone should be present there and if not, stealthily pick one up. Once in the bathroom, lock the door. The door should have a deadbolt on it. To ensure greater security, you can also plant a rubber stopper under the door. This works if the door opens into the bathroom.

Make regular bathroom sounds such as flushing the toilet or turning the water on and call for help. Call 911 and or campus police. Campus police may have the quickest response time. Calling fellow students on your cell is also an option, but only after you have called the police.

Should your date ask why you are not coming out, tell him you are sick and that he needs to go home. At that point, he will either take the advice or start pounding the door in. Should he succeed and gain entrance, your self-defense training becomes necessary.

While there are many perils associated with moving to a new location, one of the most dangerous is date rape. Statistics all prove that the incidences of this crime are higher during the college experience. Consequently, the better prepared the student is to deal with this, the greater the chance of surviving it.

Personal security expert and author of the book *How To Protect Yourself from Crime*, Ira Lipman offers this advice.

> The two most significant factors associated with campus rape are how often a woman dates and the sobriety (or lack thereof) of her date or acquaintance, as well as herself. The more men she dates, the more likely she will at some time find herself with a man with characteristics of an assailant.
>
> Also, one significant survey reported that 75 percent of men involved in acquaintance rape had consumed alcohol or drugs immediately prior to the assault. Moreover, 55 percent of the victims had consumed alcohol or drugs before the incident.
>
> If a woman does drink, she should do so in moderation and stop before she feels dizzy or high. She should find out what her tolerance is before exposing herself to potentially dangerous social situations.

Women should also keep in mind that a man's tolerance for alcohol and other intoxicants is higher than a woman's and that party environments can be ideal for the use of date-rape drugs, as well as other drugs.

Lipman goes on to list some rules to provide some protection from date rape:

- Be extremely selective in the men you date. Be aware of any signs that may signal a tendency towards assaultive behavior.

- Be on guard when dating athletes or fraternity brothers, especially during your first semester at college.

- Avoid parties where alcohol and drugs are consumed. If you must drink, know how much you can handle and observe your limit.

- Refrain from dating "macho" men who demean women.

- Define to your partner as soon as possible your sexual limits, informing him as to the behavior you consider acceptable and unacceptable. Tell him that kissing, hugging and touching are not a license for intimacy.

- Terminate your date if the man attempts any form of force or intimidation. Even if the man is a classmate or friend, unwelcome behavior is unwelcome behavior.

- Memorize the campus security or emergency telephone phone number and/or put it in your cell phone. Memorizing is good in case your cell phone is stolen. Write it down and keep it in an easily accessible place as well; if a disturbing situation develops, you may have trouble remembering it.

This is good to know should your cell phone be stolen. If you are in an area of high cell phone theft, you can always buy one that doesn't work from a resale shop and hand that off to the criminal.

- Ask a female friend or campus security officer to accompany you home after a late-night party if alcohol has made you dizzy or tired.

- Never leave a party with a man who makes sexual comments that are unwelcome or make you uncomfortable.

- If your date engages in behavior that makes you feel uncomfortable, be assertive. Tell him if he does not stop, you will end the date.

- Leave immediately with a girlfriend if you find yourself one of just a few women remaining at a fraternity party.

Lipman offers a good guide for women entering college. Nevertheless, here are additional considerations that can be addressed:

- Does the college or university have a student escort service that is accessible at night and on the weekends?

- Is there free student transportation to dormitories after dark?

- Are there realistic self-defense courses, either for credit or not, that can provide protection against potential attacks using psychological, as well as physical tactics, that the average person can do?

- Are there public phones throughout the campus that a student can call for transportation or security should she not have her cell phone with her?

- Is there a safe house for survivors of sexual assault in the close vicinity?

- Does the college or university have individuals trained in dealing with survivors of sexual assault?

Statistics regarding crime on or off campus can be found at http://ope.ed.gov/security/main.asp

STREET ASSAULTS

Street assailants generally target their intended victims by how they look as they walk. Specifically, such criminals are looking for bad posture, poor or lack of eye contact, and the appearance that a person doesn't belong or is lost. If asked a question, a potential victim turning away and/or answering softly show a lack of confidence.

To counter becoming a possible victim, do the opposite. Have good posture, return eye contact normally, answer questions assertively and be confident.

An assailant may employ so-called "boundary-crashing" tactics. He may have a map so he can ask his target a question. Another ploy might be offering to help with a package or groceries. Such inquiries split the mind of the target. Half of the mind is concentrating on the individual, while the other half is on responding to the question. Such a situation allows the assailant to get close enough to grab the victim.

Some assailants are bold enough to grab a woman walking down a sidewalk and force her between two buildings to assault her in broad daylight. Vacant buildings or areas under construction, where there is little light, can be particularly dangerous, even during the day.

If a stranger is employing boundary-crashing against you, yell "Stop!" and throw both of your hands out, as if you were throwing a basketball at the potential assailant. This is intended to shock the assailant into freezing for a brief moment.

This activity is something you can practice. In practice, the person coming toward you must have the intention of striking you or hurting you in some way. These thoughts cause tension in the body and make it freeze when you use the "Stop!" yell tactic. If there is no intent to harm, the mind will be relaxed and the shout won't work. If the person is drunk, the shout might not work, as his reflexes will be affected by alcohol as well.

If you think you are being followed, look around quickly. If you see a person move his head to the side or look down, this might be a sign that he is likely following you. If this happens on a street with retail stores, use the store windows as mirrors.

Should you notice a group of men walking toward you and your intuition is sending warning signals, when they are still about fifteen or twenty feet, slowly raise your hand, look across the street and say in a louder voice, "Hey, guys, wait up!" even if nobody is there. Then begin to cross the street. This may confuse the group walking toward you enough that they will just keep walking and not follow you.

CAMPUS DANGER ZONES

On any campus, there are areas to be wary of: dark parking garages, narrow alleys, and places where alcohol is served. For each of these locations, there is a strategy that can be adopted.

Most of all, stay relaxed and remain aware. This way, your body has a better chance of reacting to any given situation. You can induce relaxation by inhaling through your nose and exhaling through your mouth. This is especially good to do when you are exiting a location.

When walking down the street, keep to the middle of the sidewalk. This helps you avoid any attacks from an alley or from attackers in cars.

When parking your car, back into the slot with the front bumper facing out. That way, you can use the door as a shield against any attacker. If you are unable to back in for some reason, make sure you look around first to see if anyone looks suspicions or is lurking about.

Always check your surroundings for an escape route. Your chances for escape diminish when you are surrounded by walls. Any alley that has walls on three sides makes escape very difficult.

Also be aware of elevators and stairways at night. It is always a good idea to carry a tactical flashlight with you. The amount of lumens for the light should be over 120, the more lumens the better. Make sure the flashlight is easily accessible for your use. Some tactical flashlights also have a jagged bezel or edge that you can use to strike with. Or carry a small flashlight just for everyday use and one for self-defense.

Jogging can also bring with it a number of risks, including sexual assault. To minimize your risks, follow these suggestions:

♦ Jog only during daylight hours.

♦ If you must jog at night, don't distract yourself with any audio device and carry a tactical flashlight with an easily accessible strobe function.

- If attacked, strike the eyes, throat, or groin and scratch and bite.

- It is always best to take a self-defense course.

- Pepper spray or pepper gel, if easily accessible, is another option.

- If you wear a cap, use one with a metal buckle in back so that you can take it off and start striking the attacker with it.

PRACTICE AWARENESS

There are two types of awareness, *situational* awareness and *intuitive* awareness.

Situational awareness deals with your surroundings. If you need to make a 911 call, can you describe where you are? If you are running, are you heading north, south, east or west? What are the names of the streets or street numbers? What landmarks are near by?

Situational awareness also includes "people watching" and gathering information from them. If you are at a bar, check out the other patrons. A good exercise is to observe anyone who is nervous; try to figure out why. Does anyone not fit in? Is anyone wearing clothing that conceals his belt, but is continuously fussing with it, as if he were carrying a weapon. Watch the hands in this case. What kind of feeling do you get from the people close to you?

Intuitive awareness deals with your intuition. There are several exercises you can do to heighten your skill in this area. The best way to access your intuitive power is through relaxation, which you can do by practicing breathing exercises.

Breathing exercises can be done while seated or standing. If you are seated, make sure your spine is straight. If you are standing, bend your knees slightly. Then inhale through nose and exhale through mouth until you feel relaxed. Relaxation time will vary from person to person. It's also beneficial to relax before exiting a building or venue; this helps heighten your awareness and prepare for a potentially threatening situation.

If you get a feeling of danger about going into an area or about a person, heed that warning. Listen to your gut!

Also remember, consuming more than one alcoholic beverage will neutralize your intuitive abilities.

SPRING BREAK

Perhaps no other school holiday strikes students with joy and parents with fear then does spring break. An onslaught of alcohol and drugs can easily lead to rape and or kidnapping. When traveling to a spring-break location consider the following tips:

- When traveling with a larger group, book rooms next to each other.

- When going out, set a time when everyone in your group will return to the hotel—and stick to it.

- When traveling out of the country, respect local norms and dress. Do your research.

- Make a copy of your passport and keep it in a safe place. Some people have kept it in their shoe between the layer of support and the sole. Place the original for safekeeping in the hotel safe.

If you wish to have your passport on your person, get a money belt, which you can purchase at most travel stores or retailers. A money belt or pouch can be hidden under your belt or hung from the neck to go inside your blouse.

- Do not leave your purse or drink unattended when you go dancing or visit the rest room.

- Leave valuables at home.

- Use a money belt to hide credit cards and/or passport and other important documents.

- Do your best to blend in, rather then attract attention.

- If you can afford it, buy a cheap phone that you just use for travel and program it with all essential information. There are tracking services available that can track your phone in case you go missing with it on your person. Also know how to erase your personal information from your phone should it be stolen.

- Have a travel itinerary and stick to it.

- Keep your eyes open for date rape drugs. This means that you keep an eye on your friends and they keep an eye on you. Once you ingest a date rape drug, passing out is soon to follow.

- Leave your travel agenda with your parents and/or trusted friends not traveling with you.

- Avoid wearing shoes that limit your ability to run.

- If one of your friends needs to leave a party or other venue, make sure everyone goes with her.

- Check to see if your hotel has a shuttle service that will take you to a location and bring you back.

- Never keep all your money in one spot.

- If you find yourself in a robbery situation that a weapon, you can use a "drop wallet/purse" tactic. Drop the wallet/purse and run.

  A "drop purse" is a decoy in which you carry none of your essentials, because these are safely kept in your money belt.

  Another option is using your purse and keeping your valuables in the zipper compartment, in which you can keep your credit cards, passport and your serious money. You can also use a money clip. Take a lot of single bills and wrap a $20 or larger bill around them. When asked for your money, flip your purse. The valuables will stay in the purse while the money clip will drop out. Seize your opportunity to run away.

- Beware of taxis outside of the US. Research the taxi company before you travel. If possible, check if the hotel where you are staying can provide you with a shuttle. If not, check the references of the cab company you wish to use with your hotel. Why not check with the local police department? If you are unsure of the level of corruption of the location you are going to, stick with the hotel's information, as it has a vested interest in keeping you safe.

- When staying in a hotel, try to book any of the middle rooms. The first two floors are easy to break into. Being on the top floors makes you more vulnerable if a fire should break out.

- Travel with people you can trust.

RESOURCES

There are a number of non-profit organizations to address the epidemic of sexual assault on campus. For example, www.SeeActStop.org has the mission of ending sexual assault on college campuses by working with, pressuring and legislating colleges and universities to adopt best practices. These include:

- Biennial campus climate surveys with results made public
- Uniform, prompt, fair and thorough adjudications for all students, including student athletes
- Confidential advisors for survivors
- Amnesty from alcohol/drug use charges in sexual violence cases for testimony
- Anonymous reporting options
- Use of investigators with specialized training
- Alerting students that they have the right to seek outside help, including law enforcement, but are not obligated to do so.

According to End Rape On Campus (EROC), "Twenty-eight of the top 50 'best universities' in a *US News and World Report* are under federal investigation for their handling of sexual assault."

EROC's mission is to work "to end campus sexual violence through direct support for survivors and their communities; prevention through education; and policy reform at the campus, local, state, and federal levels." They can be reached at www.endrapeoncampus.org

If you are a survivor of assault, www.SurvJustice.org can offer you assistance in several ways. According to its website,

> SurvJustice increases the prospect of justice for survivors by enforcing victims' rights in campus, criminal, and civil legal systems to hold both perpetrators and enablers of sexual violence accountable. Accountability is key to decreasing the prevalence of sexual violence, which is also furthered by training institutions and supporting changemakers.

Another resource for survivors and those who wish to be active in preventing sex discrimination in schools and on campuses is www.KnowYourIX. org. Title IX is a federal civil right that prohibits sex discrimination in education. What makes this applicable to survivors is that Title IX protects any person from sex-based discrimination, regardless of their real or perceived sex, gender identity and/or gender expression. Female, male, and gender-non-conforming students, faculty, and staff are protected from any sex-based discrimination, harassment or violence.

Check to see that your school is proactive in ensuring that your campus is free of sex discrimination. It must have an established procedure for handling complaints of sex discrimination, sexual harassment or sexual violence. Your school must take immediate action to ensure that a victim can continue his or her education free of ongoing sex discrimination, sexual harassment or sexual violence.

The school may not retaliate against someone filing a complaint and must keep a victim safe from other retaliatory harassment or behavior.

Your school can issue a no-contact directive under Title IX to prevent the accused student from approaching or interacting with the victim. In cases of sexual violence, your college is prohibited from encouraging or allowing mediation (rather than a formal hearing) of the complaint. Your college should not make victims pay the costs of certain accommodations that he or she might require to continue his/her education after experiencing violence. You can find much more information at http://knowyourix.org

Another site, www.NotAlone.gov, includes information for students, schools, and anyone interested in finding resources on how to respond to and prevent sexual assault. It contains a wide variety of information

RAINN, the Rape, Abuse & Incest National Network, is the nation's largest anti-sexual-violence organization. RAINN created and operates the National Sexual Assault Hotline, 800-656-HOPE and online.rainn.org) in partnership with more than 1,100 local sexual assault service providers across the country. It also operates the Department of Defense's Safe Helpline. In 2015, the Online Hotline expanded to offer services in Spanish at rainn.org/es. RAINN also carries out programs to prevent sexual violence, help victims and ensure that rapists are brought to justice. It also has a large database on statistics, safety tips, resources for parents and friends and much more.

TEACHING BOYS TO BEHAVE

Another way to prevent sexual assault is to teach boys how to behave toward the opposite sex, and even other boys. The Centers for Disease Control (CDC) released a report in April 2014 on ways to prevent sexual assault on college campuses. It reached the conclusion that "... only three primary prevention strategies, to date, have demonstrated significant reductions in sexual violence behaviors using a rigorous evaluation methodology ... :

◆ **Safe Dates**, which is designed to prevent the initiation of emotional, physical, and sexual abuse in adolescent dating relationships.

◆ **Shifting Boundaries**, aimed at reducing the incidence and prevalence of dating violence and sexual harassment among adolescents. Intended for male and female middle school students.

◆ **RealConsent**, which is designed to reduce sexual violence perpetration behaviors among college men using a bystander-based model that draws on social cognitive and social norms theory. The goals of this program are to prevent sexually violent behavior toward women.

More information on those programs can be found at www.cdc.gov/violenceprevention/sexualviolence/ prevention.html

OTHER RESOURCES

◆ **Clerycenter.org**
This is a national non-profit organization dedicated to helping college and university officials meet the standards of the Jeanne Clery Act.

The Jeanne Clery Disclosure of Campus Security Policy and Campus Crime Statistics Act or Clery Act, signed in 1990, is a federal statute that requires all colleges and universities that participate in federal financial aid programs to keep and disclose information about crime on and near their respective campuses. Compliance is monitored by the United States Department of Education, which can impose civil penalties, up to $35,000 per violation, against institutions for each infraction and can suspend institutions from participating in federal student financial aid programs.

- **Legalmomentum.org**
  Lads action for the legal rights for women

- **Endsexualviolence.org**
  This non-profit organization provides a missing voice in Washington for state coalitions and local programs advocating against sexual violence.

- **Safercampus.org**
  This group strengthens student-led movements to combat sexual assault on campus.

- **Futureswithoutviolence.org**
  This group develops innovative ways to end violence against women, children, and families at home and around the world.

CHAPTER SIX
KEEPING YOUR FAMILY SAFE AT HOME

The media is full of reports of "home invasion." The term is actually used in a number of states to define a type of burglary. These estimates of burglary are based on a revised definition of burglary from the standard classification in the National Crime Victimization Survey (NCVS).

Historically, burglary is classified as a property crime, except when someone is home during the burglary and a household member is attacked or threatened. When someone is home during a burglary and experiences violence, NCVS classification rules categorize the victimization as a personal assault rather than a property crime (household burglary, theft, and motor vehicle theft). In this report, the definition of household burglary includes burglaries in which a household member is a victim of a violent crime. Highlights from the NCVS report include:

♦ An estimated 3.7 million burglaries occurred in the United State each year on average from 2003 to 2007.

♦ A household member was present in roughly one million burglaries, and became victims of violent crimes in 266,560 burglaries.

♦ Simple assault (15 percent) was the most common form of violence when a resident was home and violence occurred. Robbery (7 percent) and rape (3 percent were less likely to occur when a household member was present and violence occurred.

♦ Offenders were known to their victims in 65 percent of violent burglaries; offenders were strangers in 28 percent.

♦ Overall, 61 percent of offenders were unarmed when violence occurred during a burglary while a resident was present.

♦ About 12 percent of all households violently burglarized while someone was home faced an offender armed with a firearm.

♦ Households residing in single-family units and higher density structures of ten or more units were least likely to be burglarized (8 per 1,000 households) while a household member was present.

♦ Serious injury accounted for 9 percent and minor injury accounted for 36 percent of injuries sustained by household members who were home and experienced violence during a completed burglary."

(SOURCE: *U.S. Department of Justice, Office of Justice Programs, Bureau of Justice Statistics, Special Report, National Crime Victimization Survey, "Victimization During Household Burglary," September 2010 NCJ 227379. More recent editions may be available. To view a list of all reports in the series go to http://bjs.ojp.usdoj.gov/index.cfm?ty=pbdetail&lid=245).*

Thus, the bottom line is that "home invasions" are statistically rare. This doesn't mean that you shouldn't be prepared.

What if I told you that a secret weapon exists that can sense a crime before it is perpetrated? What if I told you that this weapon could even add up to two years to your lifespan, as well as help keep your family safe? Interested?

Well, the secret weapon I'm talking about isn't actually a secret. It's a guard dog. Actually, it's two guard dogs.

Professional guard dogs can be expensive, sometimes ranging from $2,500 to $45,000, so for the average family, getting a good pedigreed dog with a well-developed protective instinct, such as a German Shepherd, Doberman Pinscher, Rottweiler, Dutch Shepherd, or a Belgian Malinois, may be just the ticket.

Actually, in some cases, it's even possible to get by with just an ordinary mutt for protection purposes. When looking for a dog that will be protective of you and your family, it is good to interact with it first and get a sense of its intelligence and instincts.

> Jane was a single mom living in a second-story apartment with her son. It was after midnight when she suddenly awoke to the sounds of barking and snarling. By the time she found the reason for the disturbance, her son's American terrier was voraciously gnawing on the ankle of an intruder, who was doing all he could to get away.

When considering defending their home, most people think about installing a security alarm or buying a gun. Either of these methods, however, brings with it several potential problems.

While an alarm system can work effectively in protecting against an ordinary thief, it can be breached by an experienced career criminal. An alarm system sticker on a window, may deter entry by an inexperienced thief. However, an experienced or desperate crook knows that the police or security forces need time to get to your house. In some communities, it can also happen that the police would not respond to burglar alarms due to an overwhelming number of false alarms. In some cases, neighbors may either be too far away, asleep, or not care if your alarm goes off. In addition, some burglaries have been committed by relatives and people known by the victims.

According to Sanford Strong, a 20-year police veteran, expert in survival techniques, and the author of *Strong on Defense*,

> Eighty percent of all crime occurs in the three places where you spend most of your time—your home or adjacent to it, your place of work and its parking lot, and the public routes you travel regularly.

Armed with this knowledge, it only makes sense to develop a plan of action to accommodate these circumstances.

There are two types of home intruders: burglars and armed intruders. Burglars wait until you are gone to enter your home, which is why some people like to leave the lights on and music blaring to keep burglars out. Home intruders don't care about any of these deterrents. They'll either burst in or use some type of ruse to get you to open the door. Consequently, if you and your family find an armed intruder with a gun in your house:

- React immediately.
- Have a plan that includes a safety code word directing family members to take appropriate action, which usually means that the spouse and/or the children flee to a specified neighbor's house, while the other spouse physically attacks the intruder. It also means that one spouse may end up hurt or even dead.

Still, it's better than the other option, in which the criminal uses the threat of violence and locks up the most physically able spouse in the closet while he goes on to rape, torture, and/or kill the rest of the family. There are no perfect solutions in this scenario, and everything is situational.

- Home intruders first seek to control the adults and often do this by pointing a gun at the wife or child and making threats. If this happens, say these words with forceful intent to the intruder: "You can have anything you want in the house. But if you hurt my child or my wife, I will have nothing left to lose, and I will kill you. I've killed before, and I will do it again." It doesn't matter if you've killed or not. What matters is that the intruder doesn't know that.

- The designated family member should try to get close to the intruder to jump him. To get close to an armed intruder, ask questions that appeal to his greed and demand a response. For example, say to him, "I have a bank card. Would you like to go with me now to pull out some money?" The intruder's response will be either no, yes, or he'll ask you how much you have in the account. Either way, as you inch closer, your family can prepare to bolt when you give them an agreed-upon signal.

- While you approach, you can keep your hands up, but try to keep them under the direction in which the intruder's gun is pointing. When an intruder answers a question, about half his focus is on pulling the trigger, while the other half is on providing you with an answer.

This gives you an opportunity to move close enough to say the family code word, so that the rest of your family can bolt to safety as you jump the intruder. As to the manner of disarming the intruder, that is best studied personally under a certified instructor.

- Do not do what the intruder tells you to do. The intruder's most common method of operation is to separate the husband from his family by threatening the wife and kids. In this way, the intruder can tie the husband down or lock him in a closet. Do not let this happen.

- A good escape plan will include multiple routes to leave the house in the event the intruder has one route blocked, such as a hallway. Although not a popular choice, the spouse must decide if this is the opportunity to fight back.

- Make all your survival decisions ahead of time and practice your escape drills often with your children and spouse. Make sure everyone participates. Practice should include yelling and screaming when escaping to attract attention and discourage the intruder. Once one person has escaped the house, the intruder's will power may begin to break. In most cases, it will be a child who flees first.

- At the sound of the code word, all family members should scream and shout. Depending on the circumstances, the family member designated as the one to attack the intruder should make a decision as to whether to attack while the rest of the family escapes or escape with the family.

- Having good house lights, locks, alarms, and dogs make a huge difference.

- For second-story homes, use a knotted rope or ladder to escape through the window if necessary.

- Always have a mindset of "We will survive." You can even say this over and over to yourself when placed in dangerous circumstances.

- Breathing and relaxation are two key elements in dealing with fear, anxiety, and adrenaline. Taking breaths through the nose and exhaling through the mouth can foster the necessary relaxation.

Author Sanford Strong states that guns are by far the most ineffective weapon to have in the home as a means of defense. He points out that in America:

- Eighty-three percent of suicides by gun are committed with a firearm kept primarily for home protection.
- Ten percent of all loaded guns kept in American homes for protection end up being used to kill a family member during the heat of an argument.
- On average, one child per day is killed while playing with a loaded gun.

What is it like to be woken in the middle of the night by an intruder? Imagine suddenly waking up and finding yourself driving someone else's car on a dark country road while speeding at 75 miles an hour. You first have to find the controls and figure out how they work before you can get things under control. Now, picture yourself being awakened by an intruder in the middle of the night. You have to find your gun, unlock it, load it, and be calm enough to fire it at someone who might also be armed and fire back. Now, add a spouse and children into this deadly mix.

Despite all these factors, many people still feel it is better to have a gun. As a self-defense instructor myself, I maintain that the best solution is to make sure that you are not faced with this reality in the first place. Some precautionary measures include:

- Planting thorny bushes around your windows.

- Using a rubber door stop or an electronic one that sounds an alarm.

- Putting a baseball bat or wooden pole in the well of the patio door or sliding glass doors so that entry is impossible even if the lock is jimmied. Make sure those glass doors can withstand the force of a heavy rock being thrown at them; many burglars find such rocks in the gardens of the homes they target.

- Having bells or chimes attached to doors, or hanging above them, can make an economical burglar alarm.

- Being part of or starting a neighborhood watch.

- Getting to know your dwelling in complete darkness so you can escape without attracting attention to yourself.

- Getting a dog. Almost all dogs are watch dogs, but few are guard dogs. The difference is that a watch dog will bark, but won't necessarily engage with an intruder, while a guard dog may or may not bark, but will usually engage the stranger.

- Going through a civilian Police Academy. This is a great way to meet the police officers who patrol your area and learn what they do to keep you safe.

- Designating a safe room if your dwelling is large enough. Otherwise, consider running to a friend's house or apartment. Ideally, you should choose a location inside your apartment building or on the same street on which your house is located.

- Having well-lit corridors and parking lots if you live in an apartment building, or having motion-sensitive or light-sensitive lighting if you live in a house.

- Asking police to drive by your house when you are on vacation.

♦ Putting lights on a timer to give the illusion that you are still at home while you are away. If you go on a vacation, consider getting a reliable house sitter.

♦ Use the "Ring Video Doorbell." According to the company website:

> "Over one million burglaries occur just in the United States each year during daytime hours, when homes are usually unoccupied. Being home is often enough to deter a potential burglar. Whereas traditional security systems activate once a break-in has occurred, the Ring™ Video Doorbell is designed to help you prevent a break-in from taking place at all. Answer the door from anywhere using your wireless video doorbell. With Ring, you're always home."
> (SOURCE: https://ring.com)

Deception has always been important in military strategy, and it is no different when fighting a war on crime at home. If you, for some reason, can't have a dog, you can still create the illusion of having one by:

♦ Making sure there is a huge dog bowl outside your house with dog food strewn about it and with a name such as "Monster," "Jaws," or "Killer" written on it.

♦ Having "Beware of Vicious Dogs" signs posted.

♦ Adding a few very large deer or beef bones next to the dog dish that's outside your house is an especially good idea if you live in the country.

♦ Having an alarm that sounds like a dog barking when someone attempts to break in.

Deception techniques work best on criminals who are not from the surrounding area. Those from your neighborhood or observe your home for a number of days or weeks will see through these methods. In some burglaries, the culprit turned out to be a relative. Consequently, this brings us back to the original strategy of owning a good dog or dogs that have inherent protective instincts.

DOMESTIC VIOLENCE

> Upon reporting to 911 that her estranged husband had threatened her and was on the way to her house, Mia was informed that the police could not be sent because the restraining order she had against him had expired. Within minutes, Mia, her three children, and her estranged husband were all dead.

Mia is actually a composite of several women whose lives were destroyed by domestic violence. It is no surprise that 75 percent of spousal murders occur after the woman leaves. This makes it imperative to get out of an abusive relationship as soon as possible and more importantly, to avoid getting into one in the first place.

So how do you know if you're in a relationship with a potential abuser? Here are a few possible indicators:

- He grew up in an abusive and/or violent household.
- He can be controlling.
- He wants to accelerate the relationship into a marriage or living together commitment.
- He has a history of violent behavior.

- He uses his abuse of drugs and alcohol as an excuse for his behavior.
- He can become easily jealous of you.
- Your intuition is telling you so.

While the use of intuition can be effective, those involved in abusive relationships tend to have an intuition blackout. They tend to adopt a set of false beliefs that include:

- The abuser will change.
- The abuser is not at fault for his actions.
- They actually deserved the abuse.
- They can actually change the abuser.

Sometimes a victim's ego gets involved when she (or he) just doesn't want to admit that a wrong decision was made when committing to an abusive relationship. If intuition doesn't work, is there a way to tell if you or someone you love is in an abusive relationship? The answer is *yes* and can be found in the following quiz.

- Does your partner:
  - ☐ Want to make all the decisions for you?
  - ☐ Want to control your actions, such as who you see, where you go, and to whom you talk?
  - ☐ Want to keep you on a tight leash?
  - ☐ Limit your contact with your friends and family?
  - ☐ Take your money, make you ask for money, or refuse to give you money?

- ❏ Make you scared?
- ❏ Verbally abuse you?
- ❏ Threaten to take away or hurt your children?
- ❏ Blame you for causing him to abuse you?
- ❏ Act as though abusing you is no big deal?
- ❏ Deny abusing you even after abusing you?
- ❏ Embarrass you privately or in the company of others with putdowns or derogatory names?
- ❏ Threaten to commit suicide?
- ❏ Threaten to destroy your property or pets?
- ❏ Intimidate you with guns, knives, or other weapons?
- ❏ Shove, slap, hit, or sexually attack you?
- ❏ Threaten to kill you?
- ❏ Force you to drop charges against him?

If you answered yes to any one of these questions, you may be in an abusive relationship and require professional assistance. You can call a law enforcement agency, domestic abuse hotline, or domestic abuse shelter for help. There is also the National Domestic Violence Hotline at 1-800-799-SAFE, and if you have Internet capability, you can obtain more information from the Rape Abuse and Incest National Network (www.rainn.org) as well.

"In the United States, women are killed by intimate partners more often than by any other type of perpetrator, with the majority of these murders involving prior physical abuse," says Jacquelyn Campbell, Ph.D., R.N., author of *Risk*

Factors for Femicide. In fact, a batterer's unemployment, access to guns, and threats of deadly violence are the strongest predictors of female homicide in abusive relationships, according to a study published in the July 2003 issue of the *American Journal of Public Health.*

While there can be a long list of pre-incident indicators associated with spousal violence and homicide, the bottom line is this: ***if you don't like the relationship you are in, get help and get out.*** While you may not feel you are in danger or feel that being without your partner is worse than being with him, an objective and professional opinion has no downside. Get help, and get it now!

xxxx

CHAPTER EIGHT

WORKPLACE VIOLENCE

Is there someone at work who frightens you? Well, you might have good reason to feel unsafe.

Workplace violence costs the United States $121 billion per year, according to *Campus Safety Magazine* (November 11, 2012).

In its *2013 Workplace Violence Fact Sheet*, the National Institute for Prevention of Workplace Violence Inc. provides information, statistics and charts on workplace violence to give human resources, threat management, security, risk management and operational managers the most current information on workplace violence. Key findings include:

♦ Workplace homicides and other violent acts are the second leading cause of death for women at work.

♦ For the first 10 years of the 21st century, an average of 558 work-related homicides occurred annually in the U.S.

♦ Workplace suicides rose to an all-time high of 270 incidents in 2010.

♦ An estimated more than half million incidents reported each year most often occur in nursing homes, social services, hospitals and late-night convenient stores

♦ Non-fatal assaults alone result in more than 876,000 lost workdays and $16 million in lost wages.

♦ Subsequent costs could include lost productivity, counseling, contract/sales losses, cleaning and refurbishing, increased insurance costs, lawsuits/settlements, and more.

In its 2015 edition of *Death on the Job,* the AFL-CIO found that

> ... Workplace violence continues to be the second leading cause of job fatalities in the United States responsible for 773 worker deaths and 26,520 lost-time injuries in 2013. Women workers suffered 70 percent of the lost-time injuries related to workplace violence.

According to the report, the leading source of death from workplace homicide was assault by an assailant or suspect (211 deaths), and co-workers were responsible for 74 homicide deaths in 2013. Firearms were the primary weapon involved in workplace homicides, causing 323 workplace deaths. The leading occupations for workplace homicide were supervisors of sales workers (46 deaths), retail sales workers (43 deaths) and motor vehicle operators (37 deaths).

Retail trade was the industry with the largest number of workplace homicides in 2013 (95 deaths), followed by accommodation and food services (69 deaths), local government (39 deaths), and transportation and warehousing (36 deaths—taxi service accounted for 25 of these deaths).

Moreover, the Bureau of Labor Statistics reported that more than 26,000 workplace violence incidents led to injuries involving days away from work in 2013, an increase from 2012.

> A fired letter carrier from the post office in Dana Point, California, who had been terminated for stalking a female coworker, returned one day in December 1992, opened fire, and killed a coworker. Police later learned that the man had killed his mother prior to the shooting, shot and wounded a woman motorist shortly after it, and then shot and wounded two customers at an automated teller machine in an apparent robbery attempt.

Nearly four out of ten women killed at work are murdered. According to a report from the U.S. Department of Labor, this makes murder the leading cause of death for women in the workplace. Additionally, the National Institute for Occupational Safety and Health (NIOSH) states that since 1980, at least 750 people per year have been murdered at work. This makes murder the third-leading cause of occupational death overall. Furthermore, in the August 1994 issue of Bureau of Labor Statistics, the U.S. Department of Justice proclaimed the workplace to be the most dangerous place in America.

Although some occupations may be more inherently dangerous, one thing for certain is that workplace violence is making its presence known everywhere. Almost everyone has heard of such an incident, whether at their place of work or from the news media. It appears that there are no safe havens.

Violence has even found its way into the healthcare industry. Again, citing the Bureau of Labor Statistics, intentional injuries caused by humans, excluding self-inflicted injuries,

> Healthcare workers are at an increased risk for workplace violence. From 2002 to 2013, incidence of serious workplace violence (those requiring days off for an injured worker to recuperate) were four times more common in healthcare than in private industry on average.

The U.S. Department of Labor states that "the cost to organizations is staggering. ... a single incident can have sweeping repercussions. There can be the immediate and profound loss of life or physical or psychological repercussions felt by the victim, as well as the victim's family, friends, and co-workers; the loss of productivity and morale that sweeps through an organization after a violent incident; and the public relations impact on an employer when news of violence reaches the media ... It has been estimated that these costs could exceed $120 billion per year in the United States. "

Another survey conducted by the now-defunct National Safe Workplace Institute paints a gloomy picture. This survey revealed that out of the 248 security and safety directors questioned in 27 states, nine out of ten security directors had knowledge of more than three incidents of men stalking women employees. The survey also stated that of those surveyed, 94 percent acknowledged that domestic violence is a "high" security problem at their companies.

Information from the National Victim Center shows that for every murder, there are numerous rapes and assaults that often leave victims battered and disabled.

According to the U.S. Department of Justice, husbands and boyfriends, current and former, commit more than 13,000 acts of violence against women in the workplace every year. Additionally, statistics illustrate that 20 percent of all workplace incidents against women involving physical injury were traced to a romantic entanglement that involved either a co-worker or outside spouse or boyfriend.

In cases where there are legal injunctions or restraining orders barring perpetrators from going to the victim's home, attackers enter the workplace in their search for the intended victims. "Victims' addresses and telephone numbers can be changed, but not necessarily their places of employment" reports the National Victim Center.

WHAT EMPLOYERS CAN DO

Employers are becoming more aware of the high costs that violence can cause their companies with regard to:

- Security
- Building repair and clean-up
- Business interruptions with customers
- Lost productivity and work time
- Employee turnover
- Salary continuation for those who are injured or traumatized
- Valued employees quitting or retiring early
- Increases in workers' compensation claims, insurance premiums, and medical claims

♦ Attorney fees, medical care, and psychological care for current employees.

A company has several ways to help prevent violence. The first is by putting in place a thorough pre-employment checking mechanism. The second is by having a well-educated security force. The third is by maintaining a well-informed personnel department that encourages employee communication on these issues and sponsors programs to discuss workplace violence, including self-protection and awareness programs for its employees.

Often, too much emphasis is placed on the interview in making a hiring decision. This is because the interview is a method of determining suitability for a position and acceptability into a specific corporate culture. The potential problem with a standard job interview is that the candidate can lie, and it is very hard to determine the truth unless he or she is hooked up to a lie detector. That's why other independent means, such as calling previous employers to verify information, as well as checking on the quality of the person's character, are essential. A good pre-employment check can uncover a potential problem.

Depending on the right-to-privacy laws in each state, employers can search public records for incidents of criminal or civil misconduct. They can also access the Department of Motor Vehicles to see if the candidate's license is current and the driver is in good standing. Most records are now on computer, so checking them has become a lot easier. In fact, failure to do so may lead to accusations of negligent hiring, if something happens later.

During the hiring process, employers can also verify an applicant's social security number with the Social Security Administration to make sure he is who he says he is. Most importantly, records that list criminal convictions, judgments, liens, and civil suits are available through a number of online computer services.

Unfortunately, not every potential criminal can be screened. Employees can develop mental illnesses or suffer from depression or other stressors that can put them over the edge well after they have been hired.

While there are those who believe it is possible to compile data that identifies violence-prone behavior, the best test of violent behavior is violent behavior. If an employee stalks or threatens others in the workplace, causing them to fear him, or if there is an employee who has been written up or warned about such behavior, the employer must take immediate and appropriate steps.

Some of the best protection for an employer is to take each complaint or employee warning as seriously as possible. Intervention is the best prevention. Employers can take a number of steps to safeguard employees, as well as themselves:

- Provide on-site stress relieving services, such as offering a Pilates exercise program, massage, physical training, acupuncture, and/or counseling.

- Provide safety services, such as seminars on violence prevention or self-defense instruction.

- Provide coupons or reimbursement to employees who engage in these or other stress-relieving activities.

♦ Have a toll-free, anonymous service that employees can call if they are aware that someone is becoming dangerous.

♦ Make an effort to follow up on reports of employees who appear depressed, sullen, and/or angry, commit inappropriate acts, obsessively or romantically pursue co-workers, exhibit a fascination with violence, guns, and/or have a survivalist attitude, and make threats or behave in a threatening manner.

♦ Recognize and don't tolerate patterns of insubordination, intimidation, sabotage, threats, bullying, manipulations, and actions that cause fear and anxiety.

WHAT EMPLOYEES CAN DO

While an employer has the responsibility of keeping the workplace safe, the employer cannot do it without the help of employees. Preventing violence in the workplace is a two-way street. Employers can only act on information they receive.

If an employee feels threatened by another employee, the threatened employee must report it to the appropriate personnel. This also includes incidences of domestic violence or stalking, because when a perpetrator had threatened to follow the victim or is stalking the victim, the workplace is in danger.

If employees remain silent about their suspicions regarding another employee, they must accept the burden for whatever tragedy unfolds.

Employees can help prevent workplace violence when they:

- Report inappropriate behavior.

- Seek help for domestic abuse situations they may be experiencing, either on their own or through an employee assistance program (EAP).

- Make employers aware of potential stalking situations.

- Report incidents of suspicious employee behavior, even if it is just a "gut" feeling.

- Use an anonymous employee tip line or notify Employee Assistance or Human Resources if they suspect or overhear that a violent act may occur or that an employee has stated a desire to commit acts of violence, has obtained a weapon, is paranoid, spies on other employees, seems as though he has a huge chip on his shoulder, believes he is unfairly picked on, or is continually depressed.

- Are persistent when an employer doesn't take the necessary precautions, even if it means moving higher up the chain of command, writing and sending a certified letter to establish documentation, and, if necessary, contacting police, media, or an attorney.

- Take measures to reduce their own stress levels, which could be as simple as cutting down their caffeine intake by substituting herbal beverages for coffee or tea.

- Take care of themselves emotionally, physically, mentally and spiritually.

- Recognize that they must get professional help and get out of an abusive relationship immediately.

TERMINATION

When employers make a determination to terminate the employment of a potentially violent individual, they should:

- Not let it leak out that the employee is going to be fired. Treat the employee respectfully and do not show fear.

- Make the termination immediate so the terminated employee doesn't have to come back the next day. If the person has personal items at the workplace, allow the person to remove the items immediately. Be direct and don't lecture.

- Have security on stand by, but not necessarily in the room where the termination is to take place.

- If the employee is in sales or customer service, provide the employee some input on how to handle client calls in the future (new contact within the organization).

- Attempt to make the employee feel better by telling the individual that the job is not helping them to excel. Let the individual think he/she is a capable person.

- Terminate the employee at the end of the day when most workers on that shift have already left the place of work.

- Do not fire the employee in the employer's office, but rather, use a conference room or meeting room that offers an opportunity to leave if necessary.

- Whenever possible, have a higher-level manager with whom the employee has not worked do the firing. A second person, preferably one admired by the employee, should be there as well to help ensure that the employee is on good behavior.

- Prior to termination, depending on the conceal carry laws in your state, employers should have signs posted stating that weapons are not allowed in the workplace or in the parking lot and enforce this regulation with electronic weapons screeners.

PROFILING THE POTENTIAL FOR VIOLENCE

While there is no concrete means to identify who will get violent and when, a number of red flags can be seen as indicators. In the book, *Staying Alive*, published by Safe Havens International, Inc., the authors point to the work of doctors Stephen and Richard Holmes, who are famous for their work in forensic psychology and behavioral analysis. They identify a continuum of violence that has three levels:

- Level 1: Intimidation
- Level 2: Escalation, and
- Level 3: Further escalation

These can provide a context for a person's behavior, but doesn't mean that an individual will become violent. In their work, Holmes and Holmes state that **Level 1, Intimidation**, is the most common type of unacceptable workplace behavior. It is best to bring the following behaviors to the attention of someone who can help, like the Human Resources department.

- Refusing to cooperate with authority.
- Spreading rumors and gossip to harm others.
- Constantly arguing with others
- Making unwelcome sexual comments.

Level 2, Escalation, includes:

♦ Increasing arguments with others

♦ Refusal to obey policies and procedures.

♦ Sabotaging equipment or stealing property for revenge.

♦ Verbalizing their wishes to harm others.

♦ Sending unwanted sexual notes, emails, or tweets.

♦ Having a "me versus them" mentality.

If you are near such a person and feel threatened by that individual, there are reasons for that and you may wish to make your feelings known to Human Resources, even if it is a gut feeling. There are some people you meet whom you can't look in the eye for long without getting a bad feeling. This is another case of your intuition trying to send you a signal.

    Level 3, Further Escalation, is the most dangerous because this involves a person who already is committing violence and exhibiting frequent displays of anger, which result in:

♦ Recurrent suicidal threats.

♦ Recurrent physical fights.

♦ Destruction of property.

♦ Use of weapons to harm others.

♦ Commission of murder/rape/arson.

The best thing to do in this case is to notify the police.

PHYSICAL WARNING SIGNS OF WEAPON USE

Whether you are inside or outside a building, there are ways of identifying a person who is carrying a concealed weapon. In the book, *Scaling Force; Dynamic Decision-Making Under Threats of Violence*, Rory Miller and Lawrence A. Kane identify ways you can spot someone carrying a concealed weapon. Whereas most people who have a Carry Conceal Weapon (CCW) license will use a holster to carry their gun, criminals will rarely use one.

> The two most common ad-hoc positions for firearms are inside the pants, either in the front alongside the hipbone or in the small of the back. Because the weapon has a tendency to move around when carried in this fashion, you can often spot a bad guy touching himself to assure that it is in the proper place or adjusting the weapon to get it back into the proper carry position.

> Pants or jacket pockets are always a handy choice as well. Like the inside-the-pants carry, they are not reliable or easy to get to as a holster when you need rapid access. Weapons can also be palmed, hidden behind an arm or leg, or held out of sight beneath a covering object such as a folded jacket or newspaper. These methods facilitate rapid access but can be easier to spot then other methods. That's the good news. The bad news is that if the weapon is already drawn and held in a concealed position, you will be in extremely serious trouble if you do not spot your adversary's intent. He has already decided to attack and is moving into position to do so.

In a workplace environment, the entrance is key in identifying potential danger. There may be one entrance for employees and one for clients or one that serves both.

Ideally, there should also be security cameras placed at every entrance and exit. This, of course, varies on the size of the employer. A hair salon may not have capacity or intent to do so and in that case, the first person to make contact with someone entering the establishment is a *de facto* security agent.

If she knows the individual as one involved in a domestic abuse with a fellow employee, it is best not to confront him as he may be armed. Instead if he is asking to see his partner, acquiesce and ask him to sit down and go to a fellow employee and say "get the red folder." This is a code word to evacuate the salon and call for police.

The implementation of this strategy depends on how vocal, insistent, and demanding the abuser is. In some cases, the shooter or aggressor may go in and just start firing and in another, he will only be focused on his partner.

In either case, you will want to know if the person is armed. To this extent, the person will be exhibiting some behaviors to indicate this. The potential assailant could indeed be wearing a holster because some people licensed to carry concealed weapons have committed murder. A holstered weapon can be difficult to spot but not impossible. There are several behavioral clues to look for:

♦ Where are the person's hands in relation to his or her waistline?

♦ Are there unusual bumps or bulges?

- Is the person fidgeting with his hands trying to adjust something on their person?
- Are they wearing clothing that covers their waistline?
- Are they wearing inappropriate clothing for the weather, like a jacket, when the weather is warm?
- Is one hand resting on their jacket pocket as they walk?
- Do they look nervous and walk with an unnatural gait?

When a handgun in placed in a jacket pocket, the coat typically hangs lower on the side where the weapon is located. Other signs may include wearing a photographer's vest, or wearing a fanny pack in everyday life. Usually fanny packs are for places like fair grounds. One pant leg that tends to rise up may indicate an ankle holster. A small-of-the-back holster may be tough to spot when covered by a jacket unless the person bends down.

A greater danger exists when someone is carrying a weapon in the open, as the open-carry law allows, because you don't know if that person is a good guy or if he is looking to kill people. Open-carry activists walk around in public parks, restaurants, and other places because it is legal.

So how can you stop someone who is carrying an assault rifle when they step inside a building and start shooting? Homeland Security has a number of responses, so please follow this link: www.dhs.gov/xlibrary/assets/active_shooter_booklet.pdf.

Many of the suggestions in the Homeland Security booklet depend on timing and location. Everything is situational. A group of several people, such as in a school setting, may throw items at the shooter to activate a flinch response of the human body. It is instinctive for a person to try to avoid getting hit so he raises his arms causing his guns to point upward. That is the point where an attack on the shooter is most advantageous. People can grab the arms and tackle him to the ground and try to remove his weapons and restrain him.

Depending on where you are, running may be an option. But if you're in a room, turning your back to the shooter may lead to your possibly getting shot.

Chapter Nine
Staying Safe on the Street

I t has been said that criminals are animals. Indeed, when it comes to attacking people, they certainly can behave like animals. If you have ever seen a nature program where several lions are searching for prey, what do the predators typically seek? They look for weakest, most defenseless animal they can find. Usually, the animal is very young or old or sick, which means it cannot defend itself. This is the same behavior that most criminals look for in their victims.

Criminals are lazy. They want to choose someone they feel will be an easy victim-someone who won't fight back. Consequently, they look for someone who gives the appearance of a victim.

So what do potential victims look like? There are at least four qualities to victimhood:

1. Potential victims project low self-esteem or low energy.

2. Potential victims usually walk with their head down.

3. Potential victims seem unaware of their surroundings.

4. Potential victims communicate an attitude of surrender through their body language. When asked a question they may turn their head away or look down to try to

avoid eye contact and answer softly. They look like they won't fight back.

This falls perfectly within one part of the criminal's formula. Crimes happen when criminal intent meets opportunity. So we can say that

criminal intent + opportunity = crime.

In the Wisconsin county where I live, a woman was assaulted by a number of attackers. The incident happened in the early hours of the morning outside a convenience store in a high-crime neighborhood, which is a setting that provides criminals with the perfect opportunity to exploit the weak. As the woman left the store, they surrounded her, and one of the assailants pulled out a weapon and told her to come with them.

Unfortunately, the woman went with the assailants and was assaulted. While I cannot say whether or not she demonstrated the four qualities of victimhood, I can surmise that she was at least unaware of her surroundings, or she wouldn't have been there at such a dangerous time.

This brings me to a very important point. If anyone ever pulls out a weapon and tells you to come with them, especially after they've robbed you, don't go. After they've taken your money, the only reason they want you to move is so that they can hurt or kill you. Even before they rob you, breathe, relax, and try to get a sense of whether you can run away safely. As mentioned above, I recommend that you always carry a "drop wallet" or "drop purse" that has a lot of

$1 bills in it. If your assailant pulls a weapon, throw down the "drop wallet" and try to escape.

REFUSE TO LOOK LIKE A VICTIM

There are at least seven ways to project an "I'm not a victim" look:

1. Walk engaged. This means to walk with your head held up, shoulders squared, and with purpose.

2. Return eye contact normally. Let your eyes briefly meet to acknowledge the person coming toward you. Don't stare at the person looking at you, and don't walk looking down at the sidewalk. This may vary in large cities such as New York, where the norm is to look away.

3. Walk as though you belong. Even if you are uncertain of where you are, don't look rushed but walk at a confident and comfortable pace. Oftentimes criminals will attack you if you look lost or out of place.

4. If you're going to be out late at night or in an area with a high crime rate, don't wear anything that draws attention to you.

5. Project confidence and be aware of your surroundings.

6. Be assertive. Sometimes even a smile or nod can disarm a potential assailant.

7. If you are a senior citizen in an unsafe neighborhood, it's best not to walk alone for any length of time, especially after leaving a bank or at night. If you must walk alone, bring a pair of dogs along. Breeds that can scare an attacker away include the German Shepherd, Pitbull, Akita,or Doberman Pinscher.

Psychological Group Avoidance Exercises

It is not uncommon for someone to be walking down the street and come face to face with danger. Groups of two or more people may be looking to harass, rob, or assault victims they find on the street.

The following exercises help you develop skills to avoid such confrontations. Ideally, they should be practiced with two or more people. One person takes the role of the target while the others take the role of potential assailants.

The idea is for the target to change the focus of the assailants. Also, when faced with a group of two or more people, never try to walk through them. Always go to the side. This makes it hard for most of them to grab you. Pass close to the street. This avoids being grabbed and pushed against a building or pulled into an alley.

Exercise One

As a group approaches the target, she returns eye contact normally and smiles as he walks by. It's important not to show fear, so the target should not move more quickly than normal pace.

If the group is very close and not looking at the potential target, she should use peripheral vision to keep tabs on the group without appearing to be suspicious.

Exercise Two

This time, as a group approaches, the target looks across the street, waves his hand, and calls out, "Hey, Frank!" Of course, Frank is not there, but the group doesn't know who Frank is or if Frank is traveling with a group of friends.

While a group may take on a single target, the problems that can occur if more people get involved may keep them from acting.

Exercise Three

As the group approaches this time, the target begins a loud, disgusting cough as he walks by them. Very few people want to deal with sick individual who potentially has a communicable disease.

Exercise Four

The target approaches the group, and if he senses that the group may do him harm, he smiles and extends his hand for a handshake to the group member nearest the street. He can even say "Hi," as though he recognizes the person.

This action does three things. First, it humanizes him in front of the group. Second, it shows that he is paying respect to a member of the group. And, third, it shows that he is not afraid of the group.

As with any self-defense technique, no method works 100 percent of the time, so initially, always use your intuition when judging what action would be the most appropriate to take.

Exercise Five

This is a more advanced exercise to be practiced by couples or families. In this scenario, a family or couple is walking down the street when a gang appears. When they are within a yard or two of one another, one partner places a hand on the back of the other partner and gently directs that partner to the other side of the street.

If there are children involved, the spouse gently steers them closer to the street than she is. A split second after the movement occurs, the one partner pretends to have an untied shoelace or an ankle problem and goes to one knee. The group's focus is shifted to that partner rather than on the other and/or children.

As the group comes closer, he stands up and uses one of the previous techniques, such as smiling, and then passes the group to the side closer to the street. This splits the focus of the group in several different ways, which allows the target to walk by unharmed.

Depending on the age of the children, code words can be used to indicate a specific action to perform.

Exercise Six

This exercise deals with learning on how to spot if someone has a metallic weapon on them, like a knife or a gun. This is very beneficial to do with a group of friends you know.

Have someone bring out a metal butter knife from the kitchen. One person then takes three of your friends from your sight. He or she instructs one of the three people to take the knife and hide it on them. The person with the metal butter knife must develop thoughts about hurting the group of people, although he or she will not actually do it. The reason for this is that it will raise that person's level of tension, which may make him/her look guilty. That way, it's easier to spot the potential attacker.

The group should be seated in a way that all participants can see the three people. When the people return, they should either walk around the group or just walk in a circle in front of the group. They should walk for about one minute and then stop and just look at the group.

One person walks to the three and then places one hand above one of them and the group votes with a show of hands if that is the person with the knife. The person then goes on to do the same for the other two. Finally, after the voting, the person with the knife shows it.

The problem with working with friends is that sometimes the group knows the person who is the most likely person to carry a knife. You want to avoid this. The group should just use its intuition to select the knife-carrying person. The reason for telling the person who is to carry the knife to get those feelings of hurting people or being angry is that it causes tension in his body that can be detected by the people using their intuition.

HOW TO USE YOUR ATTITUDE TO STOP AN ATTACK

I once met a college student on a plane flight to Portland, Oregon. After brief introductions, we started talking about self-defense. She told me a chilling story about an incident that happened to her on her college campus.

One evening, she was walking from the school library to her dorm room. Suddenly, a man started to walk beside her. He said that it was dark and that she shouldn't walk alone. She said no, she didn't want him to walk with her, and continued walking. But he persisted and walked beside her, then suddenly grabbed her upper arm and began to escort her. She said nothing at this point. Noticing that he was walking slightly behind her as he held her arm, she turned around and saw that his pants were unzipped and he was behaving inappropriately. She quickly broke his hold and began to run. If it hadn't been for her sheer stamina and speed, she feels he would have caught her.

As we discussed the situation, I discovered that she never looked at her assailant—not once. When she told him no, she looked down. Her tone of voice lacked conviction, authority, and sufficient volume. When the stranger grabbed her upper arm, she didn't object because she didn't want to feel foolish.

In essence, she broke almost every rule of non-violent self-defense. She was passive. She looked away from the assailant instead of looking at him. Her tone of voice signified that she lacked authority. She showed she didn't have the confidence or the intent or the commitment to resist. She was a perfect target and potential victim, and she was very fortunate not to have been assaulted.

An attacker does not want to pick a confident woman, because he attacks to demonstrate what he believes is power and control. Because such a man is insecure, he searches for a woman whose behavior and/or actions will satisfy his needs. Therefore, an attacker is less likely to assault a woman who presents a possible challenge. He wants a sure bet.

When you convince him you are not that woman, he will look elsewhere. Carrying yourself with utmost confidence reduces your chances of becoming his victim.

In his book *Being Safe*, Dr. Edward Ross urges people to keep their head up and eyes scanning the general area where they are walking. Be attentive and alert and never underestimate any potential situation. Ross notes a recent survey of state convicts who reported that they targeted people they knew would not struggle or people they thought would not chase them after they had stolen their purse or wallet.

When asked how they picked their targets, one convict said, "I watched how they walked. If they seemed as though they had no energy and looked out of shape, they were mine." All the convicts agreed that they were less likely to challenge someone who projected a sense of confidence and self-preservation.

The same principle is true for men as well as women. Your attacker is most likely going to be bigger, stronger, faster, and meaner than you, or else he doesn't have an advantage. There are some exceptions to this rule, and they usually involve drugs and alcohol. Sometimes a blast of liquid- or drug-induced courage can cause someone to think they can do more than they can.

There are a number of categories that represent attackers. One of the most popular categories is "the bully." If you think back to the people who were bullied in your school, how did they look and behave? Why do you think they were picked on?

If you were or are bullied, ask yourself "Why?" Then ask yourself what you did or could do to prevent this. Some people might say that those who were different in some way were picked on the most. The example often cited is that of the obese child or child of smaller stature. But this may not be entirely true.

Some bullied children may not fight back, but others will. Consequently, it's not stature or obesity that is the problem, but rather an attitude of surrender. Chances are that the people being picked on were really nice people who didn't want any trouble. In other words, they projected an attitude that made them prime targets. Others who projected the intent that they would fight back probably never got picked on.

Bullies find their enjoyment in humiliating others. They are emotional vampires. Sometimes they travel in gangs, and other times they travel alone. Either way, they seek someone who is not assertive, someone who won't cause them a lot of trouble. The more isolated a person is, the better for the bully. The same behavior is sought for by the average criminal, who looks for the easy score.

This brings me back to the formula for the commission of a crime:

Crime = intent + opportunity

A criminal may have the intent to rob or hurt you, but without the opportunity, he won't do it. Part of the opportunity is the attitude of the target. Will the target be an easy target? Part of this answer lies in how you look and carry yourself. The other part lies in your attitude.

Your attitude is the way you express yourself. It is your posture and your body language. It is how you appear to others. Consequently, your attitude plays a vital role in whether or not an attacker is going to choose you. Your body language is more powerful than the spoken word. It includes your walk, posture, eye contact, facial expressions, and overall appearance. How you feel about yourself and your surroundings is reflected in how you carry yourself.

Your body language will tell others if you're strong and secure or anxious and uncertain.

A large part of your attitude in self-defense situations comes from your intent to defend yourself. You have to make a mental commitment that you will fight back if you are attacked. In certain situations, this attitude is sufficient by itself to prevent an attack.

As for the bullies, you need to fight back from the beginning. This does not necessarily mean to fight back physically. Bullies work on trying to intimidate and humili-ate you. When you resist them, you set up boundaries. And you don't have to be alone.

In the case of school bullies or relatives or employees who bully you, *complain.* You can complain to other family members or the relevant authorities. If you feel threatened, complain to the authorities. If you are in a relationship with an abusive spouse, leave and get professional assistance. Either way, you are adopting an attitude of defending yourself.

Most of the time, it is this attitude that will warn a bully or criminal not to pick on you, since they both thrive on fear. The attitude of fighting back makes the bully evaluate the amount of trouble you are going to be. Even if the bully thinks he can beat you, he may not want to try if he thinks he'll get hurt in the process.

If you are walking alone and someone pulls up in a car and taunts you, and you fear that the problem will escalate, call the police. If there aren't any stores around, say in a very loud voice, "I don't want any trouble." This will alert other pedestrians to take notice of what is going on, and it may make the bully stop the taunting. Above all, leave the scene as quickly as possible.

If, however, you are alone at night, your options may be very limited. Make smart decisions if you live in a high crime area and minimize your nighttime activities.

Also, keep in mind that not all defensive measures work all the time. Sometimes, when you have a bad feeling about a situation, you should trust it.

INTERPRETING DANGER SIGNALS

There are some concrete strategies that criminals use that we can identify in order to be safe. In *Humane Pressure Point Self-Defense*, the authors identify and condense seven signals that predict violence from Gavin de Becker's book *Gift of Fear*. They are:

1. **Forced teaming.** The assailant looks to create an attachment or partnership with the intended victim. The assailant wants to create an artificial sense of trust with the victim by being close to the victim.

2. **Charm and niceness.** These are tools the assailant may use to make the intended victim relax and let down her guard, because in our society we believe that someone who is polite and charming is a good person.

3. **Too many details.** In order to mislead an intended victim, an assailant will use "too many details" in conversation as to appear open and friendly. A skillful liar uses details to create the appearance of honesty and truth.

4. **Typecasting.** The assailant slightly insults the intended victim so that the victim feels compelled to disapprove of the accusation by cooperating with the assailant. An

example would be the assailant saying, "You're probably too snobbish to talk to the likes of me.

5. **Loan sharking.** An assailant will do an unasked for favor, such as helping the victim with groceries, as a way of making the victim feel obligated or indebted in some way or to let down their guard.

6. **Unsolicited promise.** An assailant will make an unsolicited promise as a way to reassure the victim and quiet natural suspicions. An unsolicited promise in an setting is trying to convince you to do something he wants.

7. **Discounting the word "no."** It is said of men that they take the word "no" not as the end of the discussion but as the beginning of a negotiation. If this is true of men in general, it is particularly true of assailants. This is a very important warning signal, and women would do well to learn to say the word "no" with forceful clarity. After all, many a would-be rapist has been schooled on the foul adage, "When a woman says 'no,' she really means maybe. "

Another way of predicting violence is to look at patterns. If you're in a relationship and are treated badly, but your abuser keeps apologizing, leave and seek aid from friends, family, an abuse prevention organization, or the police. Continuous abuse is a pattern, and unless it is checked, it will continue.

Other patterns that predict violence include threats—verbal or written—and stalking. If more than one negative action is taken against you, it's a pattern.

The jealous ex-boyfriend who violates restraining orders and writes or says that he is going to kill may do just that. Take action at the first instance of potentially violent behavior. Action can mean calling that police, a counseling center, and even friends or relatives. Some people buy dogs.

The advantage to having a dog is that it can sense danger before it happens, which may make a dog more efficient than a knife or gun, and, unlike a knife or gun, it can't be taken away from you and used against you. A word of caution: If the dog has been around the partner who is socialized, then it most likely won't defend you.

You can even buy a trained guard dog for further safety. The bottom line is that if you don't feel safe, you are not safe. Follow your intuition, verify the danger signals, and take immediate and appropriate action.

Fights at Bars or Public Events

Location can play an important role in the commission of a crime. Bars or public events where alcohol is served in particular have a greater chance of violence, especially for men, when it comes to fighting.

Danger signals in bars are very important to recognize, because bars are often the playground of bullies. The bar bully needs a justification to attack, as do most bullies. Usually they stare at their victim to get a response, so they can say, "Hey, what are you looking at?"

Other times, they may deliberately bump you to obtain a justification to attack you. The way to beat the bar bully on the "Hey, what are you looking at?" technique is to do either one of two things. First, ignore him until such time as he comes to you. Then, say very loudly with your hands up in the air, "I don't want any trouble!" This will attract the attention of the bartender and/or bar manager, who play an important part in this scenario, because the police usually ask the bartender or manager what he or she saw.

Another technique is to buy the bully a pitcher or drink and tell the bartender or bar manager that the bully is causing trouble. Chances are good that the bully is a regular and they will ask him to leave. That way, if an altercation occurs, the bartender can say that you purchased a drink for the bully, and then the bully went over and started trouble. This technique is for male-on-male intimidation only.

As for the "bumping into" scenario, apologize and move away. Should the bully follow, put your hands out in in front of him and yell, "I don't want to fight!" over and over while you take a step or two back. If no one interferes and you feel endangered, you may have to strike first. The impression on the patrons, though, is that you moved back, you didn't want to fight, and the bully ignored you. While this may act in your favor in a court case, it is always best to consult an attorney. In some municipalities, police no longer arrest the bar bully, but rather just ticket both parties for disturbing the peace unless someone has serious injuries.

There is also a special consideration for those partners who are with a friend, boyfriend, or husband, in a situation such as this. Do not interfere with the actions of your date or friend. If you tug at his arm or draw his attention from the bully, and if the bully is close to both of you, there is a very good chance that the bully will hit your date or friend at that moment. The best way to help is either to leave immediately to a safe place or to get the bartender or a bouncer involved quickly.

When a male is engaged in a fight with his date present, his attention will be split between the fight and the safety of his date, which could mean disastrous results for him. Both of you should practice using a code word for a specific action, which could include leaving the room or establishment, calling the police, or driving away.

In fact, it's always a good idea to see where the nearest source of help can be located, and at the first instance of a danger signal, go get help. As always, follow your intuition.

How Defensive Voice Can Stop an Attack

One should follow the principle that if one action doesn't work, you can fall back on another. Therefore, each new principle raises the bar slightly as it comes closer to potential physical violence. If one action doesn't work, you go to the next level and then to the next level, so that you have a number of principles of redundancy, the next component in your self-defense arsenal is defensive voice.

Defensive voice is a very important component when it comes to nonviolent self-defense. This technique works on a variety of levels. While many people think that it is just screaming, let me assure you that it has even more important uses and can be applied to many situations.

While many people may be familiar with the concept of verbal self-defense or verbal judo, defensive voice is much more simple and direct. Defensive voice is focused mostly on tone. It's how you say something. Both men and women can use defensive voice and may use it in different applications.

Simply put, your "defensive voice" is a short sentence spoken in a commanding tone and often giving an instruction.

For instance, let's begin with dating. Whether you are dating or your daughter is dating, this technique may prove invaluable.

If your date makes improper advances and you want him to stop, treat him as though he is a dog. By that, I mean you have to issue commands.

Making elaborate explanations as to why you don't want to do something with your date may only challenge your date to overcome these defenses. It can become a competition that ends very badly for you.

So keep your commands short, as you would if you were talking to a dog. You wouldn't tell a dog that you really feel it should stop what it is doing because it's inappropriate. Instead, you would shout "No!" or "Stop!" or "Go away!" Do the same thing with your date. Men are used to hearing commands and take them more seriously.

I use the word "command" because it signifies a specific tone of voice. If you demurely and softly say the word "no," it will have no power. You have to use the appropriate voice for your commands. That's why, if you visualize you're talking to a dog, you are more likely to get the correct tone.

Sometimes it may be a relative who is giving you trouble, for instance a "drunken uncle." You can use the same strategy. Being assertive and using defensive voice may help to control the situation.

Now let's move it up a notch. You meet a charming stranger, and he offers to help you with something, but the little voice in your head tells you there is something wrong. Don't say, "It's all right. I can manage." Instead, in your clear commanding voice, say, "No, go away!" In some cases, swearing at them can help, as some men grew up knowing they could get away with anything as long as their parents didn't swear at them.

This last scenario is often called the interview phase, because the assailant interviews the victim to see if she will fight back or not. Another term used is "boundary crashing," as the assailant tries to get close to you as much as possible to grab you. Yell "Stop!" or "Halt!" while throwing both palms out. This should stop his advances and give you time to escape.

Defensive Voice for Men

A man's defensive voice can come in a few variations. First, there is the use of humor. For example, tell him, "I don't want any trouble. I have a bad back, but a good attorney." Humor tells the attacker that you may not be afraid of him. It may make the potential attacker think twice. While he's distracted, walk away.

When faced with the potential for a fight, the target should raise his arms with palms out to the potential attacker and yell in a loud, clear voice, "STOP!" This does two things.

First, yelling sends the alert for help, if there are people nearby. Second, your posture and your voice continuously saying this may make the attacker self-conscious enough to stop his actions. Your physical posture may also make an attack less likely because the attacker may have a hard time getting an opening for a strike, especially if you put your hands up and start moving them around as you walk away.

THE ATTACK PHASE

Whether you are a man or a woman, there are common strategies you can employ when attacked physically in public. First, notice if there are any people around. If so, identify one by what he or she is wearing and call to them for help. Specifically, you can say, "Hey, you in the red jacket and blue jeans, call the police" or "Help me now."

People who have been selected in this manner may have a higher predisposition to call for help on your behalf, especially if there are other people around and they start to stare at the identified person. You don't have to stop at identifying just one person either.

> Samantha, who worked at a check cashing business, had attended one of my women's self-defense workshops. One night, she was followed to her residence by two masked men in a van. As she left her car, one of the masked men grabbed her arm. She quickly made a defensive move she learned at the seminar and freed herself. She then noticed the other man with the gun. She quickly created distance and started calling for help. Her neighbors opened their windows to see what was going on. Some of them shouted, "We're calling the police!" At that point, the two masked men jumped in the van and sped off.

Samantha's tactics worked partially because there were people around. But what if you're all alone? As mentioned earlier in this chapter, there is the use of intuition and psychology. To this, add the commonsense advice of not going to high-crime areas, especially at night. Avoidance is your best defense.

Still, crime can occur when we least expect it. If one has discounted all the warning signs, forgotten to use the methods mentioned earlier in this chapter, and is physically attacked, the recourse with the most success, according to Edward N. Ross, Ph.D., is to fight back (see the next chapter).

ARMED ROBBERY

The response to someone holding a gun on you and asking for your money is quite simple. Give it to him. If you wish to minimize your losses, carry a drop wallet stuffed with one-dollar bills or play money, as mentioned at the beginning of this chapter.

Depending on the situation, and if you are more than a few feet away from the criminal, you can throw the drop wallet to the ground and run. This maneuver doesn't guarantee that you won't be shot, but the greater the distance you create, the less the chance of becoming a fatality.

In those situations where you comply and give the criminal your wallet, he may ask you to come with him. This is bad news, because the primary reason for this action is usually to hurt or kill you. Your only recourse here might be to try to run away. While physically fighting back is a possibility, unless you've had realistic training in gun disarming, it may not be your best option.

> When Cindy was in high school, she was working in a pro shop on a golf course when a robber approached her. Frightened, she emptied the cash register for him. He then told her to go with him to the back room, where the safe was kept. He told her to open it, and she did. He then took the contents and left.

In this scenario, the robber was clearly only interested in the money. Cindy complied and was not hurt. Some businesses use safes with timers, or they post video cameras or post signs that the clerks do not know the combination to the safe. This, however, may not stop a criminal from reaching over to grab cash from the register.

In retail establishments where only one person is working, hiring security personnel or the use of bulletproof glass and doors can be a lifesaver. The clerk, too, can use his intuition and call the police if he feels there might be some danger. Even if no explicit criminal activity has taken place, he can still request a squad car to come. It won't be with red lights and siren, but at least the clerk knows that help is on the way should there be any criminal activity.

If the retail establishment is in a high-crime area, the police should make a number of visits to it anyway, and the owner of the business should request it. The stronger the potential target is, the less desire there is to attack it. There are exceptions to this rule, such as when a criminal is under the influence of drugs or alcohol and doesn't have the reasoning capability to make this determination.

For those working in high-crime areas, wearing a bulletproof vest can be a life-saver. The price of the vest varies according to the its ability to stop certain kinds of bullets. Bulletproof vests can cost less than guns and be more practical.

REDUCING ROAD RAGE / AGGRESSIVE ACTIONS
In today's society, incidents of road rage are becoming more common. What makes road rage unique is that it often isn't done by professional criminals. Almost anyone can commit road rage given the sufficient amount of stressors in his or her life. Consequently, your response may need to take this into consideration.

The key to handling a road rage situation lies in knowing how road rage works and when you will be physically attacked. It is also important to consider that while we call outbursts of anger and violence "road rage," they can occur off the highway as well.

One of the biggest causes of violent behavior is stress. Whether it's the stress from work or the stress from being fired from work or the stress from a school environment, some people internalize the stress and then blow up. One parent killing another parent over a child's hockey game is a good example.

While you cannot compel others to practice some type of relaxation method to help deal with their stress, you can take one yourself. Ways of reducing stress include swim-ming, massage, Tai Chi Chuan, Chi Kung, deep-breathing exercises, acupuncture, acupressure, Pilates, meditation, yoga, walking, spending time with supportive friends, and even ballroom dancing. The key to obtaining success in these practices is to make them a part of your life routine.

Deep-breathing exercises can relax you and help you stay calm and focused. Breathing is simple. You can go to a quiet undisturbed place, sit down, and just breathe naturally. Listen to yourself breathe. The ability to relax can also help you deal with the stress of an attack. Even sitting quietly and undisturbed with your eyes closed for 30 minutes can make a world of difference.

As discussed above under the section on workplace violence, employers would be wise to offer some of these practices at work. Workplace violence U.S. employers about $120 billion per year, according to the National Institute for Occupational Safety and Health (NIOSH). Stress is the biggest cause of violent behavior, whether it is the stress from work, being fired, or from a domestic situation.

If you are confronted with someone coming at you in a rage and yelling at you, do not respond likewise. This is not the type of situation in which you use defensive voice. What you want to do in this situation, if you can't get away from the person, is to engage the person in conversation and keep the person talking. You should be calm, and your voice should be relaxed. Try to keep a distance between you and the other person, even if this means raising your hands as I mentioned previously, only this time, use a low, calming voice, almost a whisper.

When you notice that the person's sentences are growing shorter or he's just using a word or two, this may indicate that he is about to strike. If you can, take a step or two back and try to keep him engaged in the conversation. Do not get angry, because this may give him the psychological reason he needs to strike at you. Stay calm and act as if you are trying to understand and help him.

Often these situations occur before you have time to take out a cell phone or summon help, so reassuring the person that you have his best interests at heart may be your ticket to avoiding a violent reaction. If you suspect he may attack, leave as soon as you can.

TAKE ACTION

Everyone has the right to be safe. Unfortunately, in many areas of the country, personal safety is practically nonexistent. While politicians and pundits often make careers by blaring the "be tough on crime" mantra, they typically ignore the factors that cause crime to occur in the first place.

Principally, crime thrives in areas of high poverty. There is a reason that is significant number of violent crimes with firearms are committed by young males under the age of 21. Specifically, a combination of poor educational opportunities, joblessness or jobs with lower wages, and underpaid and overworked parents who can't spend quantity and quality of time required to positively impact a child's life.

Picture a young man in this type of environment where his choice is to work (if work is available) at a low-paying, dead-end job or deal drugs with the accompanying delusion of making quick money without suffering any negative consequences. For some young men, it is safer to live in jail than in their own neighborhoods. Consequently, the idea of spending time in jail is not a deterrent.

Another factor in the increase in arrests is the lack of proper policing, or overly aggressive policing in high-poverty areas. Higher crime areas demand a higher level of police presence. In many cities, however, there is talk about using surveillance cameras rather than beefing up the police force, despite the fact that there's little evidence that this is effective. Great Britain, which has one of the highest concentrations of surveillance cameras, has unfortunately not been able to prevent terrorist attacks. The police officer remains as the best sentinel in the war on crime.

Being smart on crime means that citizens should have a greater focus on the community policing model and request greater police presence in higher crime areas. In addition, there should be a concerted push for politicians and the business community to bring jobs that pay a livable family wage and provide affordable health care to those who live in higher crime areas.

ANGER

Being safe on the street has a new impediment. It is anger. More people are becoming victims of violence due to anger. Anger is rapidly replacing drugs as the reason for violence. Falling mostly in the domain of young males, this type of violence comes from arguing, showing disrespect and the poor choice of ego over common sense. While these incidents usually are trapped in the areas of lower income, the potential exists for it to spread to shopping malls and other areas of public commerce.

While we can look at societal issues for some causes to anger, we cannot ignore individual responsibility. Consequently, if you or someone you know has a short temper, look to ways of curbing it through meditation or relaxation techniques. Outbursts of anger can also occur in individuals who are taking steroids. Often referred to as "Roid Rage," its effects can lead to disastrous results for the user and the people in his life.

SMART ON CRIME

The bottom line is that we're all in this together. If we ignore the plight of those less fortunate, sooner or later it will affect us all. Likewise, if we ignore the symptoms of violence in us or those we love, we will become affected by them. Stopping street violence means finding methods to prevent crime from occurring, such as working to reduce poverty, using treatment modalities for first-time minor drug offenders instead of incarceration, taking responsibility for our own actions.

Chapter Ten
Preventing Sexual Violence

S exual assault is a form of sexual violence, as is rape. Some of the best ways to prevent sexual violence lie in knowing who is likely to attack you, where you are likely to be attacked, what age groups are most vulnerable to assault, the time most attacks occur, whether weapons are used, and the type of actions that can halt an attack.

Statistics from the U.S Bureau of Justice show that someone is sexually assaulted in America every 98 seconds. On average, there are 321,500 victims (age 12 or older) of rape and sexual assault each year in the United States. Please keep in mind that statistics can change with each study. As mentioned above, RAINN regularly updates statistics on sexual assault victims. Here are some of the numbers cited by RAINN, based on Department of Justice and the National Crime Victimization Survey, 2010-2014 (2015).

- Approximately 66 percent of rape victims know their assailant.
- 93 percent of juvenile sexual assault victims know their attacker.
- 34.2 percent of attackers were family members.
- 58.7 percent were acquaintances.

- Only 7 percent of the perpetrators were strangers to the victim.

- For 80 percent of juvenile victims, the perpetrator was a parent. 6 percent were other relatives. 4 percent were unmarried partners of a parent. 5 percent were "other" (from siblings to strangers).

- 48 percent are raped by a friend.

- 30 percent are raped by a stranger.

- 16 percent are raped by an intimate.

- 2 percent are raped by another relative.

- 4 percent are unknown.

STATISTICAL BREAKDOWN BY AGE OF THE VICTIM

- Ages 12-34 are the years of the highest risk, with girls age 16-19 being four times more likely than the general population to be victims of rape, attempted rape, or sexual assault.

- 80 percent of victims are under the age of 30.

- 44 percent are under 18.

- 29 percent are age 12-17.

- 15 percent are under age of 12.

STATISTICAL BREAKDOWN BY LOCATION

- About 4 out of 10 sexual assaults take place at the victim's home.

- About 2 out of 10 take place at the home of a friend, neighbor, or relative.

- About 1 in 10 takes place outside, away from home.

- About 1 in 12 takes place in a parking garage.
- More than half of all rape/sexual incidents were reported by victims to have occurred within one mile of their home or at their home.

STATISTICAL BREAKDOWN BY THE TIME

- 43 percent of rapes occur between 6pm and midnight.
- 24 percent occur between midnight and 6am.
- 33 percent take place between 6am and 6pm

USE OF WEAPONS IN THE COMMISSION OF RAPE

- About 11 percent of rapes involved the use of a weapon (6 percent used a gun, 4 percent used a knife, and 1 percent was some other weapon).
- Personal weapons, such as hands, feet, or teeth were used in two out of three cases of sexual assault.

The Bureau of Justice Statistics (BJS) reports that the majority of rapes and sexual assaults perpetrated against women and girls in the United States between 1992 and 2000 were not reported to the police. Only 36 percent of rapes, 34 percent of attempted rapes, and 26 percent of sexual assaults were reported to law enforcement officials.

While the Hollywood version of this crime typically depicts a stranger jumping out of the bushes, the sad fact is that most women are assaulted by someone they know as an acquaintance. This means that as soon as you feel uncomfortable with anyone (it doesn't matter who), speak up, Say no, use defensive voice, and if it is an authority figure, call a rape crisis center and/or the police.

It is important to set your boundaries, be assertive, and fight back. If you are in an abusive relationship, leave. There are many counseling centers you can call to assist you as well as the police. If you are uncomfortable about a situation at work, tell your employer. Depending on the size of the company, employers usually have a human resources department or an employee assistance program you can contact. If it's a small company, talk to the owner of the company. Under the legal doctrine of respondent superior, the employer has an obligation to provide you with a safe working environment.

In crimes of sexual violence, assailants act as most criminals do. Prior to an attack, most assailants check out their victims ahead of time. This means that the person you feel staring at you probably is. In addition to the danger signals I mentioned earlier, there are three steps that an attacker uses to check out a potential victim, especially a potential victim whom the attacker does not know.

- **Step 1:** The attacker checks for vulnerability. Are you alone? What is the physical proximity? They pick someone to whom they have access. This may occur in both stranger and acquaintance situations.

- **Step 2:** Testing the target. This is where the attacker takes a low commitment behavior from which they can easily back off to figure out what you are going to do. They want to get a feel for whether you are vulnerable or not, so they may approach you to see what you are going to do. Are you going to act passively to the overtures they are making? If so, that tells them you are the person they are after.

However, if you act assertively and establish a boundary and call them on their boundary crashing, you are giving them a signal that this might be too difficult. In a majority of cases, the attacker will back off.

♦ **Step 3:** Locking in on you as a target. The assailant has made up his mind to attack you. So now he wants to scare or intimidate you. At this point, you still have your verbal and assertive strategy that you can use, such as defensive voice. This scenario may vary in an acquaintance situation, where the attacker wishes to cajole the victim more to get what he wants rather than act physically.

Either way, tell the assailant in a clear and commanding tone to stop what he is doing or to go away. Do not act afraid as this is what they are after. Do not act indecisive, even though you may have a relationship with this person. The bottom line is for him to follow your commands. Have a cell phone handy and call the police if necessary.

Another option that people feel is viable prior to an actual struggle is running. But there are a number of potential problems with this action. First, remember that the person attacking you is usually going to be bigger than you are. So if you run, he may catch you. Second, if you are in a relationship with the person, he may just call you over and grab you without giving you a chance to run.

As always, assault is a crime of intent and opportunity. You may be on a bed or sofa or at a party and psychological-ly you don't want anyone to know what's going on because you are in a relationship with this person. You want the other person to stop what he is doing, but you don't want to injure the other. What can you do in these situations?

Obviously, the first thing is to avoid such as situation. However, if you cannot avoid it, there are a number of things you can do. If you are attacked, fight back, More and more evidence is mounting that fighting back is beneficial to stopping an attack. Also, running is not a bad idea, but you should first surmise if you can outrun your attacker. If not, then hurt your attacker first, so he can't run after you.

People generally don't grow up wanting to hit someone or getting hit themselves, so resisting an attack can be psychologically difficult. This may be especially true if the person attacking you is someone you know and trust as an acquaintance. Therefore, there are two ways you can fight back physically when all other techniques have failed.

The first is to fight naturally, which means gouging, scratching, punching, biting, kicking, and just plain going crazy on him. Focus on the vital points of the attacker—the eyes, throat, and groin. The eyes can be most vulnerable when you can poke, jab, gouge, or scratch them. Make sure that you have intent and will follow through on your defenses and combine your attack with yelling or screaming.

As for the acquaintance assault, you can choose the same strategy, but oftentimes people hesitate to follow through because it's someone they know. If the person has not heeded your defensive voice and tries to attack you, use the same strategy as above. Always think: *I will survive.* Still, your best bet is obtaining self-defense training from a qualified instructor.

Carrie was barely five feet tall. A young mother, she has just put her baby daughter to bed when she heard a noise. She first tried to ignore and reason it away. After all, she lived in a very small town where crime rarely happened. Still it, nagged at the back of her mind.

She didn't have to wait long to discover what the noise was. With one thundering crash, her screen door hit the floor and a total stranger landed in her kitchen. No words were exchanged as the large man grabbed and threw her down. Carrie hit the ground and froze, not knowing what to do.

Just then her baby let out a cry. Although she had been petrified, the baby's cry turned her into a ferocious tiger. Her assailant was twice her size, but she fought back with a fury. She managed to get up from the floor. The attacker, obviously angered, picked her up as though she was a rag doll and threw her into the wall and then ran away. She recovered quickly and went to her baby.

Clearly, Carrie's attacker could have won the fight physically. He could have assaulted or killed her, and yet he chose to run away. When I first heard this story, it reinforced my belief that criminals want an easy prey. Once the prey begins to put up a struggle, there comes a point in the assailant's mind when his course of action just isn't worth pursuing. I call this "the flight point," The assailant makes a concrete decision to run away.

Additionally, according to Edward N. Ross, Ph.D., in his book *Being Safe*, major research on rape avoidance and survival shows the following.

- Women can and do deter rape even in situations where resistance appears to be futile.

- Successful resistance can occur regardless of age, ethnicity, education, or lifestyle.

- Most types of resistance proved to be effective in some manner, such as calling a neighbor, making noises, or engaging revolting behavior.

- Forceful resistance, using physical aggressiveness with or without a weapon, was more likely to provoke attack or injury, but those who resisted were less likely to be raped.

- The more strategies that were combined, such as physical aggression with screaming and yelling, the higher the likelihood of avoiding rape.

- Fleeing or attempting to flee was the most effective, but least frequently used, strategy.

- The most frequently used strategy—talking—was ineffective to deter a rape. Pleasing was ineffective as it acknowledges the rapist's power and domination, as well as the woman's submission, thereby increasing the determination to rape. Crying was also mostly unsuccessful.

- All women who did nothing to resist were raped.

- Women who acted immediately, aggressively, and vigorously were the most effective in resisting rape. Initially, aggressive victims were found to be twice as successful in warding off a rape as those who were not.

- Some of those who described feeling enraged toward their attackers for even thinking of raping them were able to avoid rape.

- In spite of offering no resistance at all, some victims were kicked, slapped, and punched, as well as raped.

CHAPTER ELEVEN
DEALING WITH AN UNCOOPERATIVE, VIOLENT FELON

Pam ended up getting a divorce from her abusive husband, Gary, who went to jail on felony charges. While some would say that his going to jail appeared to be a happy ending to what had been a horrible relationship, a significant problem occurred when the time to parole Gary drew near.

Gary was a chameleon. He played the model prisoner, but in fact, he violated the law while in prison by contacting people who had a restraining order issued against him.

Pam was very concerned for her safety and the safety of her loved ones, because Gary had threatened to kill her numerous times before he got locked up. She even believed that he could have people spy on her and report back to him.

What could Pam do to stay safe? In this particular case, she was dealing with a felon who was not being cooperative. However, his infractions of the law had not been reported because Pam was unsure of what to do and was scared. Fear can cause one to withhold proper action from taking place.

In a situation where a dangerous person is about to come up for parole, there are a number of steps that can be taken.

PRE-RELEASE PHASE

The following actions may be taken to increase the chance of your safety while the felon is still in prison.

1. A letter detailing his violations can be sent to the Department of Corrections.

2. If a restraining order is issued against an ex-husband, the former wife may qualify for certain state-run victim assistance programs. Calling your state Attorney General's office or even your local state representative will provide some answers.

3. Call the local or surrounding police department and join crime stoppers. They can provide additional information on staying safe, and in some cases they do a free security evaluation of your premises.

4. At anytime you feel that any state office is not cooperating sufficiently with you, give the governor's or the lieutenant governor's office a call.

5. If necessary, consider changing your name and social security number and relocating. This may sound drastic, but when faced with the possibility of death coupled with the lack of support from your state or from within your community, it may be the logical choice.

6. Take a reality-based self-defense course as soon as possible.

RELEASE PHASE

1. If the ex-husband is getting out soon and the political resources are not able to help sufficiently, send letters to the press making them aware of the situation. This may create enough pressure to keep the eye of law enforcement officials on him.

2. Obtain a certified guard dog or two to be kept in the house. This is one of the best defenses there is. Make sure that the dog is obtained from a certified and reputable institution. Professional guard dogs can be expensive, but so can purchasing and placing intruder alarms through the house, which is another option. However, if the dogs currently in residence know and like the felon, they will be of no use.

3. Make your employer aware of the situation. Also request that the hours of employment can be varied so as to prevent stalking.

4. Avoid going to the typical entertainment venues and hanging out at the same places, especially if those are the places that were frequented with the ex-husband.

5. Make your local police department aware of the circumstances.

6. Make Crime Stoppers aware of the circumstances.

7. Carry a cell phone and learn to use the video portion of it. A number of apps allow you to make recordings. Please check with your state as to what is legal to record between parties. This helps establish evidence in case of a stalking or a violation of a restraining order.

8. Have the security guard at your workplace escort you to your vehicle.

9. If you sense or believe you are at risk, call and go immediately to a shelter.

10. Attend a civilian police academy course, if the city offers one.

PROBATION

While Pam's situation dealt with someone about to be paroled, there are also measures that can be taken when an individual is on probation. Specifically, individuals on probation are assigned a probation officer, which is usually a state function. If the felon is uncooperative, his probation officer must be notified, as well as the police.

Not all recommendations fit every situation. Rural areas do not have as many resources as urban areas do. Consequently, moving out of a location may be the only choice some people have. The important thing is to take action. When a person announces that they are going to kill someone, they eventually will. Proper action must be taken and taken immediately.

CHAPTER TWELVE
TERRORISM:
FOREIGN, DOMESTIC, AND STOCHASTIC

News headlines are full of the graphic details of terrorist attacks overseas, and even on our own home soil. Many people are very concerned about these incidents, and vigilance is recommended no matter where you travel or live.

There is also a difference between a terrorist attack to kill as many people as possible and an attack by foreign kidnappers to extort money. According to multiple sources, countries with the highest amount of danger for tourists include Mexico, India, Columbia, Haiti, Guatemala, Afghanistan, Mali, Egypt, Somalia, Honduras, Iraq, North Korea, and Sri Lanka. For the latest alerts and warnings go to http://travel.state.gov/content/passports/en/alertswarnings.html

Using numbers from the Centers for Disease Control and Prevention (CDC), from 2001 to 2014 (the most recent data available), 440,095 people died by firearms in the United States, including homicide, accident, and suicide. The U.S. Department of State reports that the number of US citizens killed overseas as a result of terrorism incidents in that same time frame was 369. If the number of terrorism incidents on US soil, 3,043 people were killed in domestic acts of terrorism, totaling 3,412.

For every one non-military American killed by an act of terror in the US or abroad in 2014, more than 1,049 died because of firearms.

Nevertheless, there are ways terrorist acts may be thwarted. From Gavin de Becker's book *Fear Less: Real Truth About Risk, Safety, and Security in a Time of Terrorism*, come these suggestions regarding airplane flights:

- Have bathrooms built within the cockpit space for pilot use only.

- Stop the in-flight meal service for pilots and, instead, stock the cockpit with preflight meals and drinks, because the meal service provides the most substantial advantage to hijackers.

- Fabricate and install cockpit doors that are bullet resistant.

- Install a locking system that makes the door's entry resistant.

- Install a system that allows officials on the ground to monitor the sounds in the cockpit if there is a loss of radio contact or the plane is off course.

- Have a video and audio system that allows pilots to observe and listen to the area outside the cockpit.

- Make cockpit security part of preflight instructions with words to the effect that protection of the cockpit door is the duty of both crew and passengers.

- Require pilots to keep cockpit doors closed at all times when there are passengers onboard.

I would add that there should be increased security checks for pilots, cargo, and crew of private corporate airplanes.

De Becker, a specialist in security issues, also contends there are steps that you can do as a passenger:

- Pay attention to anything that triggers your intuition, such as two people who aren't traveling together, but who seem to be communicating in some way; people who are adjusting items under their coats; people who seem uncommonly anxious; and people who are suspicious in ways that you can't even explain.

- Terrorists, much like predators in nature, look for the easiest kill. Once airplanes beef up security, they move on to other forms of transportation, such as buses, ships, and trains. What can be done to keep these potential targets safe?

- Encourage airlines to provide separate and bomb-proof compartments for luggage.

- Create a separate transportation system to carry luggage only.

- Create smaller passenger train cars to limit a bomb blast.

- Use bomb-sniffing dogs at travel stations.

- Run security checks on applicants for driving trucks that transport deadly cargo, including gasoline.

- Have resources available to check the cargo of ships at all our ports of entry.

Beyond these practical recommendations, de Becker offers sage advice in dealing with fear.

- When you feel fear or any intuitive signal, listen.

- When you don't feel fear, don't manufacture it.

- If you find yourself creating worry, explore and discover why."

DOMESTIC TERRORISM

According to the June 24, 2015 *New York Times* article entitled "Homegrown Extremists Tied to Deadlier Toll Than Jihadists in U.S. Since 9/11:

> Since Sept. 11, 2001, nearly twice as many people have been killed by white supremacists, antigovernment fanatics and other non-Muslim extremists than by radical Muslims: 48 have been killed by extremists who are not Muslim, including the recent mass killing in Charleston, S.C., compared with 26 by self-proclaimed jihadists, according to a count by New America, a Washington research center.

In fact, You are more than seven times as likely to be killed by right-wing extremists than by Muslim terrorists.

The attack in the Charleston church where African-Americans were attending was done by an avowed white supremacist who has since been convicted. This is only one of a number of attacks conducted by people who espouse racial hatred. Some of these groups deny the legitimacy of most statutory laws. Assaults have taken the lives of police officers, random civilians as well as members of racial and religious organizations.

In 2012, a neo-Nazi named Wade Michael Page entered a Sikh temple in Wisconsin and opened fire, killing six people and seriously wounding three others. Mr. Page, who died at the scene, was a member of a white supremacist group called the Northern Hammerskins.

In another case, in June 2014, Jerad and Amanda Miller, a married couple with radical antigovernment views, entered a Las Vegas pizza restaurant and fatally shot two police officers who were eating lunch. On the bodies, they left a swastika, a flag inscribed with the slogan "Don't tread on me" and a note saying, "This is the start of the revolution." Then they killed a third person in a nearby Walmart."

A 2009 report by the Department of Homeland Security, which warned that an ailing economy and the election of the first black president might prompt a violent reaction from white supremacists, was withdrawn in the face of conservative criticism. Its main author, Daryl Johnson, later accused the department of "gutting" its staffing for such research.

One organization tracking hate groups in the US is the Southern Poverty Law Center. The SPLC is the premiere U.S. non-profit organization monitoring the activities of domestic hate groups and other extremists—including the Ku Klux Klan, the neo-Nazi movement, neo-Confederates, racist skinheads, black separatists, anti-government militias, Christian Identity adherents, and others. They are currently monitoring around 1000 such groups across the country. They also publish reports on these groups. Their website is www.splcenter.org

STOCHASTIC TERRORISM

Stochastic terrorism is a new danger Americans face. Most people are not familiar with it. It is the use of mass communications to stir up random lone wolves to carry out violent or terrorist acts that are statistically predictable, but individually unpredictable.

In Daniel Jonah Goldhagen's book, *Hitler's Willing Executioners,* labeling a group of people as "vermin, mongrels, life unworthy of life, subhumans, etc.," were the names the Nazis used to dehumanize the Jews. Goldhagen attributes this stochastic terrorism as the main tool used by the Nazis to recruit their willing executioners.

How is this tactic being used today? One could refer to the killing of George Tiller, the Kansas abortion doctor and what FOX News host Bill O'Reilly said about him. He referred to Tiller twenty-eight times. Here are some of his comments. He repeatedly referred to the doctor as "Tiller the Baby Killer:

- "If you want to kill a baby, you hire Tiller. You've got to pay him $5,000 up front, and he'll kill the baby."

- "No question Dr. Tiller has blood on his hands."

- "Dr. George Tiller destroys fetuses for just about any reason, right up until the birth date."

- "This man executes babies that are about to be born."

- "This is the kind of stuff happened in Mao's China, Hitler's Germany, Stalin's Soviet Union."

Remember, the person who actually kills the public official, doctor, or police officer, is not the stochastic terrorist; he is the agent set in motion by the stochastic terrorist. The stochastic terrorist is the person who uses mass media as his means of setting those killers in motion. By preaching intolerance and hatred against an individual or group, the stochastic terrorist rallies forces, some of which may be emotionally unstable, but have access to firearms, to seek his own brand of justice.

On July 27, 2008, Jim David Adkisson walked into the Tennessee Valley Unitarian Universalist Church and shot nine people, killing two and wounding seven. Adkisson stated he was motivated by hatred of "Democrats, liberals, n -----s, and faggots." A police search of his home found books by Michael Savage, Sean Hannity, and Bill O'Reilly.

On April 4, 2009, Richard Poplawski shot five Pittsburgh, PA, police officers, leaving three dead and two seriously wounded. According to people who knew him, he was a birther and white supremacist, was paranoid that President Obama was going to take away his guns, and was consumed with anti-Semitic conspiracy theories. A police search of his computer found links to various groups and to a YouTube video of Glenn Beck talking about FEMA concentration camps.

On July 18, 2010, Byron Williams set out from his mother's home in Groveland, CA, heading for San Francisco to shoot up the Tides Foundation and the ACLU, with the intention of "starting a revolution." Williams, who is a convicted felon, was stopped by the California Highway Patrol (CHP) for weaving in and out of traffic at high speed. When stopped, he immediately opened fire on the CHP officers, wounding two. They returned fire and wounded him. They found the notebook in his car, with the details of his plans.

The danger of stochastic terrorism lies in its current invisibility to the general public. You could be going to work or to a hospital or house of faith and not know that someone in the media with whom you are not familiar or have not listened to, has targeted that the place you are going to.

One of the ways to deal with this is to return to the fairness doctrine. Before the dawning of hate or shock media, there was a law that called for equal representation on the airwaves called "The Fairness Doctrine." This was a policy of the United States Federal Communications Commission (FCC) introduced in 1949 that required the holders of broadcast licenses to both present controversial issues of public importance and to do so in a manner that was—in the Commission's view—honest, equitable, and balanced." In other words, if a person with one political viewpoint was on the program, you were supposed to have someone on with the opposite perspective. This was to ensure that the American people would be given both sides of an issue to make an informed decision.

Additionally, the rule mandated that broadcasters alert anyone subject to a personal attack in their programming and give them a chance to respond, and required any broadcasters who endorsed political candidates to invite other candidates to respond. The FCC began to reconsider the rule in the mid-1980s, and revoked it in 1987. With the rule gone, broadcasters were allowed to offer only one viewpoint and even lie and influence their followers, which led to extreme polarization. The current debate about climate change is a good example of this.

CHAPTER THIRTEEN

GUN VIOLENCE IS KILLING US

Oone night, you have a dream and in this dream, you do not need to have a license to drive a car, nor registration, nor insurance, nor pass any tests, nor have any training and in some states even children can handle a car. These laws were all taken away because they inconvenienced the good drivers. Wouldn't you say this dream is more of a nightmare? Well, replace the word "car" with "gun."

There are more than thirty thousand deaths per year due to gun violence each year. The US clearly leads all industrialized nations in deaths by gun violence. According to an article on January 12, 2015 in *The Atlantic* by Adrienne LaFrance,

> For the better part of a century, the machine most likely to kill an American has been the automobile. Car crashes killed 33,561 people in 2012, the most recent year for which data is available, according to the National Highway Traffic Safety Administration. Firearms killed 32,251 people in the United States in 2011, the most recent year for which the Centers for Disease Control has data.
>
> But this year gun deaths are expected to surpass car deaths. That's according to a Center for American Progress report, which cites CDC data that shows guns will kill more Americans under 25 than cars in 2015. Already more than a quarter of the teenagers—15 years old and up—who die of

injuries in the United States are killed in gun-related
incidents, according to the American Academy of Pediatrics.

Data from the CDC states your chances of being a victim of a
criminal with a gun are .0001%. However, if you keep a gun
in your home, you are 22 times more likely to become a
victim of a gun crime, suicide, or accident. It also makes
your home a target for robbery.

While these statistics are horrific by themselves, keep
in mind they do not cover those injured by gun violence
who may have their whole lives ruined. Nor do they cover
the medical coverage and associated costs that these
victims must have. According to an April 17, 2015 article by
the Law Center To Prevent Gun Violence, researchers
conservatively estimate that gun violence costs the American economy at least $229 billion every year, including $8.6
billion in direct expenses, such as for emergency and
medical care. Gun violence costs more than $700 per
American every year, more than the total economic cost of
obesity and almost as much as the annual price tag for the
entire Medicaid program.

Half of these costs are borne by U.S. taxpayers. But
these costs are not borne evenly. Data shows that states
with smart gun laws save lives and funds. Wyoming, with
the nation's highest rate of gun deaths, also bears the
highest gun violence costs per capita of any state: gun
violence costs Wyoming around $1,400 per resident every
year, twice the national average.

By comparison, Hawaii and Rhode Island have the
nation's lowest rates of gun deaths and costs associated

with gun violence of $234 per resident per year, about one-sixth of Wyoming's.

Aren't we supposed to be really worried about terrorism? According to the Global Terrorism Database, 3,521 Americans have died from terror attacks in the United States since 1970. Gun violence, on the other hand, has taken more than twice as many lives—8,512—in 2015 alone.

Mass shootings are now becoming more common, according to the Harvard School of Public Health and Congressional Research Service. In fact, they have tripled since 2011. Between 1982 and 2011, mass shootings occurred every 200 days, and between 2011 and 2014, they occurred every 64 days.

Discussions on gun violence can be volatile and arguments can be deliberately misleading due to the passions and amount of misinformation flying around, so we need to know exactly what we are debating and what is true. Here are some of the most common claims made by those who do not wish to have any laws or restrictions placed on gun ownership.

Since the late 1970s, there has been an organized effort to use access to firearms as a political issue with one side crying that the other would take their guns away. No only has this not happened, but laws have actually become more lax. How can we best decipher the facts from the fiction?

The answer comes in the source material. What is that? It is information from scientific bodies. Global warming is a good example. Almost all top scientists agree that it is real and man-made, yet there are those who don't believe in climate change because of propaganda being manufactured by those interests that stand to lose money if there are tougher regulations.

Speaking of misleading information, in 2015, the website www.beliefnet.com caused a stir on social media with an entry entitled, "Harvard University Study Reveals Astonishing Link Between Firearms, Crime and Gun Control." The post pointed to a "virtually unpublicized" 2007 paper by Don Kates and Gary Mauser that uses international data to argue that higher rates of gun ownership correlate with lower crime rates.

According to Evan Defllippis and Devin Hughes in an October 21 article in *The Trace*, "... the phrase 'Harvard study' is a misnomer, as the paper was not written by researchers affiliated with Harvard University. Kates is a prominent, NRA-backed Second Amendment activist, while Mauser is a well-known Canadian gun advocate. Their paper appeared in the *Harvard Journal of Law & Public Policy*, a journal that, unlike most academic publications, does not have peer review. The publication describes itself as a "student-edited" law review that provides a forum for "conservative and libertarian legal scholarship."

The journal's past contents include a thoroughly repudiated article, "What is Marriage?" which argued that gay marriage was morally wrong. One function that publications like the *Harvard Journal of Law & Public Policy* serve is to provide a home for papers that wouldn't survive vetting by other academics. Research that can pass peer review is almost always sent to publications whose more stringent standards also come with greater reach." The bottom line is that honest debate and truth may be a casualty when arguing gun violence.

Predictably, the strongest argument put forth by the gun lobby side is that contained within the Second Amendment of the U.S. Constitution. Specifically, the Second Amendment reads, "A well-regulated Militia, being necessary to the security of a free State, the right of the people to keep and bear Arms, shall not be infringed." It sounds pretty simple and for about 218 years, judges overwhelmingly concluded that the amendment authorized states to form militias, or as we now call it, the National Guard.

In 2008, in the case of District of Columbia vs. Heller, an opinion of the U.S. Supreme Court written by Justice Antonin Scalia declared that the Constitution confers a right to own a gun for self-defense in the home. Still, that decision allows for some restrictions. You can't own bazookas, for example. However, it is easy to get military-grade ammunition and firearms.

In a *U.S. News & World Report* dated July 24, 2014, Michael Waldman, president of the Brennan Center for Justice at the NYU School of Law, commented on what changes occurred and how in the Heller case.

> So when did the idea of an individual right to gun ownership begin to take root?
>
> There were plenty of guns in the founding era, and people expected to have the right to defend themselves, especially in their homes. But there were also many gun control laws. For example, it was illegal to keep a loaded gun in your home in Boston at the time they ratified the Second Amendment. But then the militias faded away; the

country changed. It grew more individualized. People had plenty of guns as the country spread west. Again, there were always gun laws. And the Supreme Court stayed out. The courts never interpreted the Second Amendment as reflecting an individual's right to gun ownership in two centuries.

What spurred the Supreme Court to rule as it did in the Heller case? What changed was a very successful, long-running constitutional campaign by the National Rifle Association (NRA) and its allies. They worked hard to change the way the public and the courts saw the Second Amendment and what it meant.

For a long time, the NRA was a group focused on marksmanship training, speaking for hunters and sportsmen. Then, in the 1970s, it moved very aggressively toward a more doctrinaire view and recast itself as [being on] a constitutional crusade. It worked to change public opinion about what the [Second Amendment] meant. It worked to change what the agencies of government thought. By the time the Heller case came up before the Supreme Court, it fell like a ripe apple from the tree.

Why do I state that there are limits to trying to interpret the framers' intent? Justice Scalia called the Heller case the "vindication" of his philosophy of originalism—the idea that the only legitimate way to look at a constitutional provision is to ask what it meant to the framers. In my opinion, that's really not the right way to understand the Constitution. In Heller, I suggest Justice Scalia skipped over the motivating force behind the Second Amendment. Only two pages out of his 64-page opinion dealt with the militias, which was what the entire debate in the House of Representatives was about. Yes, it's important to understand the original meaning and the text. That said, it's also critical to understand how the country has changed and evolved.

Why has it been so difficult to pass gun legislation in Congress? NRA members and gun rights supporters are very passionate and will vote for candidates based just on their stance on this issue. It's that passion rather than money that has been the source of their power.

There are numerous common-sense laws that could make a difference that don't come close to touching on the Second Amendment: stronger background checks, technological fixes to make it harder for children to accidentally fire weapons, or smart guns, which recognize their owners. But I worry that Second Amendment fundamentalism—which says that anything touching on guns at all violates a sacred individual right—could derail the kind of innovation that could make a big difference.

In the Sunday, July 2, 2017 edition of the *New York Times*, an article by Pulitzer prize-winning author, journalist, and historian Garry Wills on the Constitution appeared with a clear interpretation of the Second Amendment and its true intent. "The Second Amendment ... was not meant to let individuals prevent federal 'tyranny'—how could it? By training our rifles or handguns on the army, navy, and air force? It was meant to guarantee the legality of a 'well-regulated' [that is, state-controlled] militia to handle the states' internal problems, especially the problems of a large slave population."

THE MOST POPULAR PRO-GUN VIOLENCE ARGUMENTS

The *"good guy with a gun"* argument says that we need more good guys with guns to stop bad guys with guns. Let's take a closer look at this statement. What it says is, if there are ten kids on a playground and one of them has some stones and starts throwing them at the other kids, as a parent or teacher, you don't take those stones away from him, but rather you give stones to the other kids.

In a July 12, 2013 article in the *Milwaukee Journal-Sentinel*, two "good guys" engaged in a gun battle due to a road rage incident. They are called "good guys" because they both had legal conceal-carry permits. It doesn't mean that they won't kill anyone.

In the October 26, 2015 issue of *The New York Times*, the editorial board had this to say about concealed carry,

> The more that sensational gun violence afflicts the nation, the more that the myth of the vigilant citizen packing a legally permitted concealed weapon, fully prepared to stop the next mass shooter in his tracks, is promoted.' 'This foolhardy notion of quick-draw resistance, however, is dramatically contradicted by a research project showing that, since 2007, at least 763 people have been killed in 579 shootings that did not involve self-defense.

> Tellingly, the vast majority of these concealed-carry, licensed shooters killed themselves or others rather than taking down a perpetrator. The death toll includes 29 mass killings of three or more people by concealed-carry shooters who took 139 lives; 17 police officers shot to death, and—in the ultimate

> contradiction of concealed carry as a personal safety factor—223 suicides.
>
> Compared with the 579 non-self-defense, concealed-carry shootings, there were only 21 cases in which self-defense was determined to be a factor. The tally by the Violence Policy Center, is necessarily incomplete because the gun lobby has been so successful in persuading gullible state and national legislators that concealed-carry is essential to public safety, thus blocking the extensive data collection that should be mandatory for an obvious and severe public health problem. For that reason, the Center has been forced to rely largely on news accounts and limited data in 38 states and the District of Columbia."

The argument that *conceal-carry weapons (CCW) reduce crime* implies that gun violence would go down if we have more people carrying guns. The Violence Policy Center analyzed news reports and found that CCW permit holders have killed at least 14 law enforcement officers and 622 private citizens since May 2007. These incidents include 27 mass shootings and 39 murder-suicides.

On Monday, June 26, 2017, law enforcement officials and community leaders hosted a town hall meeting to discuss violence in Milwaukee, Wisconsin. The panel included Police Chief Ed Flynn, and the audience was able to submit written questions for the panel. The police chief was asked whether Wisconsin's concealed carry law contributes to the violence in our cities.

He stated, "It's an irresponsible law passed by irresponsible legislatures who are more interested in ideological points and I'd sure as hell like some more community outrage about that because that's what driving the violence in this city and too many public officials are silent on it."

The president of the Milwaukee Police Association took issue with these comments and said, "I have never had a conversation with you, Chief, relative to your displaying that we are arresting an overwhelming amount of people, or even one person, who's committed a crime while carrying a CCW (permit,)"

Flynn's response to this statement was chilling. "I am forbidden to tell the public when a CCW-permit holder breaks the law. I'm forbidden by statute."

If CCW was working, we wouldn't need a law to prevent the people from knowing that. In fact, isn't it true that one would only need such a law if it is a failure?

Additionally, Stanford Law School Professor John Donohue found that states that adopted right-to-carry laws have experienced a 13- to 15-percent increase in violent crime within ten years after enacting those laws (June 21, 2017, *Stanford News*).

Details on these incidents can be found at www.concealedcarrykillers.org

According to another report by the Law Center to Prevent Gun Violence posted on September 10, 2015, "A *Los Angeles Times* analysis of Texas CCW holders, for example, found that between 1995 and 2000, more than 400 criminals—including rapists and armed robbers—had been issued CCW licenses under the state's permitting law.

> A similar study by the *South Florida Sun-Sentinel* found that people licensed to carry guns in the first half of 2006 in Florida included more than 1,400 individuals who had pleaded guilty or no contest to felonies, 216 individuals with outstanding warrants, 128 people with active domestic violence injunctions against them, and six registered sex offenders.
>
> An investigation by the *Indianapolis Star* regarding CCW permit holders in Indiana revealed similar problems with the state's permitting system."

Another gun argument that follows along the lines of CCW is the **open carry opinion**, which says people will be safer if there are more guns on the street. In my opinion, this is false.

In an article written by Jesse Paul in the *Denver Post on* November 3, 2015,

> Naomi Bettis told the *Denver Post* she called 911 after spotting her neighbor, 33-year-old Noah Harpham, armed with a rifle on the street. She says a dispatcher explained Colorado allows public handling of firearms. Harpham went on to kill three people...
>
> In Denver, police say they always respond to reports of a person openly carrying a firearm because doing so is banned in the city.

According to WSB-TV in Atlanta, Georgia, a story posted April 24, 2014, led with the headline, "Man with gun causes scare during children's baseball game." The report reads:

> Parents at a Forysth County park abruptly stopped a children's baseball game after growing suspicions of

the behavior of a man carrying a gun in a waist holster Tuesday night.

"He's just walking around [saying] 'See my gun? Look, I got a gun and there's nothing you can do about it.' He knew he was frightening people. He knew exactly what he was doing," said parent Karen Rabb.

Rabb told Channel 2's Tom Regan the parents grew so alarmed that they brought the game to a halt when the man declined a request that he leave a parking lot overlooking the baseball field.

"He scared people to the point where we stopped the game, took the kids out of the dugout and behind the dugout, and kind of hunkered down," Rabb said. Park users flooded 911 with 22 calls about the man. Forysth County deputies questioned the man, and found that he had a permit for the handgun. Authorities said since the man made no verbal threats or gestures, they could neither arrest him nor ask him to leave the park."

"When I was reading my son's story last night, he turned to me and said 'Mommy, did that man want to kill me?'" said Rabb.

The *"More gun regulation leads to taking guns away"* argument says that any restriction on guns is a step closer to confiscation. This is like saying any restrictions on cars bring people lead a step closer to confiscation. There are many restrictions in place on how vehicles are produced and operated. No one argues for confiscating cars despite arguments offered to make cars safer. Also, being able to legally drive a car requires testing, having a license, and holding insurance.

Almost every time one hears of a mass shooting, the mental health argument pops up. It's not lax gun laws that are to blame; it's mental health. Apparently, then, the U.S. is the only country in the world that has mental health issues. The fact is that other industrialized countries also have mental health issues, but have in place stricter gun laws that don't allow easy access to guns by those with mental illness.

Most everyone is familiar with the *"guns don't kill people, people kill people"* argument. So if guns don't kill people, why do the military and police have them? Easy access to guns allows for mass shootings. Mass shootings and murders are a lot easier with guns, as happened at Sandy Hook Elementary School in 2012. One cannot kill 20 children in a matter of seconds with a knife.

If we made guns harder to get, bad guys and evil doers would still have them because they don't obey the law. So in other words, don't make rape laws tougher because criminals will not obey them. Don't make drunk driving laws tougher because drunk drivers won't obey them.

The truth is that in states and industrialized countries that have stricter gun laws, there is less gun violence. Europe, Australia, and Japan don't have as much gun violence. Could we aspire to this status as well?

For instance, while Switzerland has higher gun ownership than its European neighbors, it also has stricter gun laws then the U.S. Swiss law also requires that all men serve time in the military; those who do are therefore armed. Once the soldiers leave the military, they have to apply for a permit to possess a firearm.

Let me comment on the *"Background checks don't work"* argument. In 1998, as part of the Brady Act, the FBI created the National Instant Criminal Background Check System, known as NICS, which aggregates state and federal criminal databases. The law requires that every time a firearm is transferred between a federally licensed dealer and a customer, the customer fills out the form, the dealer calls the NICS phone center and gets approval for the transaction.

Among the criteria that makes someone ineligible for gun ownership: having a criminal record, specifically for felony convictions or violent misdemeanors, such as domestic abuse, as well as being deemed mentally ill by a court; or being involuntarily committed to a mental health facility; or being in the United States illegally.

Please keep in mind that laws can change and what is illegal one day might be legal the next. That said, this law applies only to *federally licensed dealers*. No background checks are required for private gun sales (at least not at the time this book was being written.)

Data from the FBI shows that each year, approximately more than 70,000 potential gun owners fail background checks, which means that firearms do not fall into the wrong hands. However, since not all purchases are through federally licensed dealers, there is no way to know how many guns fall into the wrong hands.

If a background check takes the FBI longer than three days to complete, a gun dealer can sell the gun anyway. This is how Dylann Roof, the 2015 Charleston church shooter, acquired a gun.

Another argument: **"Background checks are inconvenient and why should good people be inconvenienced?"**

For the same reason good people have to pass a driver's test to drive a car. In fact, it takes more time to get a driver's license than it does to get a gun. What we're talking about here is filling out a form that includes 16 questions relating to the potential purchaser's background, drug use, and criminal history. From its inception in 1998 through the end of 2014, NICS processed a total of 202,536,522 transactions, 1,166,676 of which have been denied, or fewer than 6 percent.

Another popular argument used to smear common-sense gun laws is that *"the blank (fill in the gun law) law would not have stopped this particular shooting."* This may or may not be true, but it would have stopped another shooting and that is the point.

WHAT ABOUT GUN-FREE ZONES?

Gun-free zones are more dangerous because most shooters target gun-free zones. No data exists that states that the shooters specifically chose gun-free zones. For example, take the man who opened fire in a Sikh temple in Milwaukee, Wisconsin, in 2012, killing six people.

Are we to believe that a white supremacist targeted the Sikh temple because it was a place that didn't allow firearms or because it was filled with members of a religious minority he despised?

In the March 25, 2015 edition of *USA Today*,

> Among the 62 mass shootings over the last 30 years that we studied, not a single case includes evidence that the killer chose to target a place because it banned guns. To the contrary, in many of the cases

there was clearly another motive for the choice of location.

For example, 20 were workplace shootings, most of which involved perpetrators who felt wronged by employers and colleagues.

Last September, when a troubled man working at a sign manufacturer in Minneapolis was told he would be let go, he pulled out a 9mm Glock and killed six people and injured another before putting a bullet in his own head.

Similar tragedies unfolded at a beer distributor in Connecticut in 2010 and at a plastics factory in Kentucky in 2008. Or consider the 12 school shootings ..., in which all but one of the killers had personal ties to the school they struck. FBI investigators learned from one witness, for example, that the mass shooter in Newtown had long been fixated on Sandy Hook Elementary School, which he'd once attended.

HAVING A GUN LICENSE ALLOWS TRACKING

Here's another argument: having a gun license allows bureaucrats, the state, and the government to know who has guns so they can take them away later. There is no evidence that the government has ever taken guns away from any law-abiding citizen. There is also no evidence that they plan to. This argument is like saying having a car license means the government knows you have a car and can take it away from you even if you have done nothing wrong.

MORE GUNS, LESS CRIME

As gun sales increase, crime falls. This is a rather dishonest argument because instead of using the term "gun violence," which is what is at issue, the term "crime" is used. The difference is that crime includes gun violence, but also includes all other crimes. Thus, while gun violence may be prevalent, it is eclipsed by all other criminal statistics to minimize how awful it can be. In other words, when we talk about gun violence, we don't care if the amount of pick pocketing has fallen.

GUNS ON COLLEGE CAMPUSES

Recently, gun-lobby-supported politicians have been trying to get guns on college campuses because somehow getting guns into the hands of college students who have the opportunity to binge drink makes everything safer. One student commented that gun bans "effectively disarm students" and puts them at risk.

The statement regarding gun bans is patently false. First of all, students are not banned from owning guns, just from bringing them on campus. In states where gun laws have become lax, gun violence has increased, so to say stricter gun laws put students at risk is deceptive. Again, why then do countries that have stricter gun laws have less gun violence than we do.

SENIORS AND GUNS

Seniors are not exempt from hearing how having a gun will protect them when the "bad guy" has a gun. The thought behind this statement is that when your physical abilities fail, a gun can help you.

There are several problems with this argument. First, if your physical abilities begin to fail, it also means your accuracy, judgement, vision, timing, and strength are impacted. Second, if we had stricter gun laws, the bad guy would not be able to access that gun so easily.

Kids and Guns

There are two issues going on when we talk about kids and guns. The first is the easy access to guns, which makes the United States number one in the world of people being killed by kids. The second is that whittling away at existing hunter safely laws to expose kids to guns as soon as possible.

The gun lobby would like to get our children exposed to guns at as young an age as possible to get them hooked. Gun proponents try to do this by offering what are called "safety" classes. There is no reason children should be exposed to guns in school. The best safety class is telling your child not to touch a gun and call for help.

With regard to the first issue—easy access to guns—lax gun laws have made it easier for youngsters to get hold of firearms. We do not have a national law that details how guns should be stored. We do not have a uniform policy on how to hold accountable people who make it easy for children to obtain guns.

In an article written for *The Trace* on April 12, 2016, she states, Kate Masters states,

> In late March, a Tennessee House committee
> defeated "MaKayla's Law," a bill that would have
> made it a crime to leave a loaded firearm

unattended and readily accessible to a child under 13 years of age. The legislation was named after MaKayla Dyer, an eight-year-old girl who was fatally shot by an 11-year-old neighbor in the hamlet of White Pine.

Before the shooting, MaKayla had refused to let the boy play with her new puppy. That's when he went to an unlocked closet, retrieved a loaded shotgun, pointed it through a window at her, and pulled the trigger.

As lawmakers in Nashville considered the measure, the National Rifle Association emerged as one of its most outspoken opponents.

"If anti-gun legislators were serious about keeping kids safe, they would know that the key to reducing firearm accidents isn't about prosecuting after the fact," reads an alert issued by the NRA-ILA, the group's lobbying arm."

The National Rifle Association (NRA) touts its "Eddie Eagle" program, which they say is designed to help prevent such accidents. In an article published in *Pediatrics* magazine, the official journal of the American Academy of Pediatrics:

> The group claims the program has helped lead to an 80 percent reduction in fatal firearms accidents involving children. But research paints a much different picture: Two separate studies of Eddie Eagle, both published by *Pediatrics* in 2004, found that the program is ineffective at teaching children how to safely respond to an unsupervised firearm in a real-life situation.

In his book, *The Last Gun: How Changes in the Gun Industry Are Killing Americans and What It Will Take to Stop It*, Tom Diaz states,

> But not everyone agrees that kids and guns don't mix. Gun-rights activists, with the help of the NRA and blinkered judges have relentlessly pushed back the boundaries of common senses to ensure their "right" to bring their guns to their children's Peewee football, Little League baseball, and soccer games, not to mention public parks, bars, churches and schools.

A CNN report on May 4, 2017 by Jen Christensen stated that according to the most recent data from 2012 by the Agency for Healthcare Research and Quality Healthcare Cost, and the Project Kids' in-patient database, 16 children per day, or 5,862 children per year, were hospitalized due to firearm injuries.

GUNS AND MASS SHOOTINGS

A study conducted by Frederic Lemieux, professor and program director of the Bachelor in Police and Security Studies; Master's in Security and Safety Leadership; and Master's in Strategic Cyber Operations and Information Management, at George Washington University on mass shootings, indicated that this phenomenon is not limited to the United States.

> Mass shootings also took place in 25 other wealthy nations between 1983 and 2013, but the number of mass shootings in the United States far surpasses

that of any other country included in the study during the same period of time.

- The US had 78 mass shootings during that 30-year period.

- The highest number of mass shootings experienced outside the United States was in Germany – where seven shootings occurred.

- In the other 24 industrialized countries taken together, 41 mass shootings took place. In other words, the US had nearly double the number of mass shootings than all other 24 countries combined in the same 30-year period.

Lemieux also states:

> In most restrictive background checks performed in developed countries, citizens are required to train for gun handling, obtain a license for hunting or provide proof of membership to a shooting range.

> Individuals must prove that they do not belong to any 'prohibited group,' such as the mentally ill, criminals, children or those at high risk of committing violent crime, such as individuals with a police record of threatening the life of another.

> Here's the bottom line. With these provisions, most US active shooters would have been denied the purchase of a firearm.

In fact, it is easier to buy a gun then it is to rent an Eddie Eagle costume, as Samantha Bee found out in this clip. http://mediamatters.org/video/2016/04/12/samantha-

bee-shows-how-easy-it-s-easier-buy-gun-without-
background-check-rent-nra-s-eddie-eagle/209874

WHY SO MANY SHOOTINGS?

It is no surprise that seldom a news cycle goes by without
the report of a shooting or mass shooting. How did we get
here? Apparently, the gun lobby has developed a strategy
by watching what had been happening to the tobacco
industry. The tobacco industry had a chokehold on Congress, but when data started to arrive from the Centers for
Disease Control (CDC) that showed how harmful smoking
was, Congress enacted the Tobacco Control Act. It led to
Americans smoking fewer cigarettes.

Josh Israel, in his December 1, 2015 article entitled
*"The Gun Industry Has Systematically Demolished Regulators
And Avoided The Fate of Cigarettes,"* activists used five ways
to hold Big Tobacco accountable for lying about the dangers
of smoking. They pursued the legal process and reached a
settlement in 1998 that involved 46 state Attorneys General
and the four largest tobacco companies, which ultimately
paid out hundreds of billions of dollars to the states and to
end many of their marketing tactics. The settlement went
on to establish the Truth Initiative to use public education
to reduce smoking among youth and young adults.

GUNS AND POLITICS

The same fate of lawsuits awaited the gun industry. In 1999,
the Clinton Administration joined the efforts with HUD,
vowing to pursue a lawsuit against the firearms industry on
behalf of public housing authorities. The gun lobby fired

back, stating this was harassment. In 2000, Smith and Wesson agreed to a settlement and promised to provide safety devices, limit magazine capacity, cut off dealers and distributors who had a history of selling to criminals, and prevent authorized dealers from selling at gun shows where any arms sales are permitted without a background check.

The NRA quickly decried Smith and Wesson's common-sense response and set out to punish it. Using the American Legislative Exchange Council (ALEC), the NRA pushed through the "Defense of free Market and Public Safety Resolution" to hurt Smith and Wesson's ability to sell to law enforcement.

Lisa Graves, Executive Director of the Center for Media and Democracy, stated, "ALEC helped to try to punish the one component of the industry that agreed to these measures," discouraging local police from buying guns from Smith and Wesson—for daring to go along with safety measures designed to keep kids safe.

With the election of NRA's candidate, George W. Bush, the new HUD Secretary quickly ended the lawsuits. In 2005, Bush signed a law that effectively shielded the gun industry from legal liability when its products are used in criminal and unlawful ways, called the "Protection of Lawful Commerce in Arms Act."

While in the past, organizations like the National Institutes of Health, did extensive research on tobacco and its harmful affects, the NRA has successfully lobbied and stopped similar research on gun violence. In 1996, the NRA and Rep. Jay Dickey, (R-AR) pushed though the Dickey Amendment, which stated that no funds "made available for injury prevention and control at the Centers for Disease Control and Prevention may be used to advocate or promote gun control." Similar restrictions were placed on NIH funding for that year, too.

WHY AREN'T GUNS TREATED LIKE CIGARETTES?

We are all aware of smoke-free zones and smoke-free-air zones. We don't hear any controversy about that because we know that second-hand smoke can hurt or kill us. Yet mention gun-free zones and the NRA launches its objections.

The NRA has fought to make sure that students can carry guns on college and university campuses. It has been a successful strategy, as now there are only about eight campuses that oppose such permissions.

ALEC is working on those eight through a model bill for state legislatures called "Campus Personal Protection Act."

Never mind that adding guns to a binge drinking environment with a high sexual assault rate is like pouring gasoline on a fire and saying that the gasoline will put out the fire.

However, the NRA doesn't see it that way and has made statements that it is the gun-free zone that is to blame. That statement has been proven to be "largely false" by a 2012 *Mother Jones* article about mass shootings.

SHOULD TAXES BE RAISED ON NON-HUNTING FIREARMS?

A tactic that may work in decreasing gun violence is increasing taxes. It is a strategy that has had some success in reducing smoking. The NRA has denounced this idea as "misguided and burdensome" and ineffective penalties on "law-abiding gun owners," rather than criminals who "don't legally purchase firearms." Unfortunately, some law-abiding gun owners go on to commit gun violence.

By the same token, financial incentives could be provided to states to mandate child-proof or personalized guns, according to data provided in *Reducing Gun Violence in America,* edited by Daniel W. Webster and Jon S. Vernick.

A comprehensive analysis by Mayors Against Illegal Guns found that most guns used in recent mass shootings were, in fact, purchased legally. Conservatives tend to denounce "big" government, except when it comes to guns. Through something called "preemption," the gun lobby and ALEC have gotten several states to pass laws that block local governments from enacting any local regulations relating to firearms.

GUNS AND DOCTORS

Perhaps no conversation can be more sacred than that of doctor and patient, but that hasn't stopped the gun lobby from pushing for legislation that prohibits doctors from bringing up the issue of guns with their patients.

"While the conversations doctors have with patients about smoking relate to cessation and the ones they have about guns relate to safety, the Law Center to Prevent Gun Violence's Laura Cutilletta says they are no less important.

> According to one study, 64 percent of individuals who received verbal firearm storage safety counseling from their doctors improved their gun safety practices....

> ...It's not about having guns. It's about storage. How is the gun stored? Is it in a home with children? Loaded or unloaded? Locked? Is ammunition stored separately?
>
> Those are the kinds of questions doctors can ask and talk about.

But, with the support of the NRA, Florida's legislature passed legislation in 2011 to chill even those conversations. The "Privacy of Firearm Owners Act" serves as a statewide gag rule, prohibiting doctors in the Sunshine State from bringing up guns with their patients. In addition to insisting that "inquiries regarding firearm ownership or possession should not be made," the law also prohibits the medical community from discriminating against patients on the basis of "firearm ownership or possession" — affording gun owners a public accommodation protection the state does not even afford LGBT people—and allows for disciplinary action of doctors who violate its provisions."

Through these actions and with the help of their allies like ALEC, the gun lobby has eliminated the tools, once used by tobacco activists to inform the public about the dangers of smoking, so that the American people are and continue to be deprived of the knowledge about the dangers of gun violence.

How Can We Solve America's Gun Violence Problem?

So what are the solutions to curbing gun violence? There are a number of industrialized countries that have stricter gun laws. The challenge comes with balancing the law so citizens can have access to guns, but the society can be safe from gun violence. To have a fair comparison between countries, let's take a look to our neighbor to the North, Canada.

Considering gun homicides in Canada, we find that in 2013, 131 people were killed. In the same year in the US, 11,000 people were killed.

Why such a difference? One can point to the fact that Canada does not have a gun lobby like the NRA, which in 2014, spent over $32 million dollars in the political arena to get what it wanted.

How about gun ownership? Canada ranks thirteenth in the world in gun ownership, with 30.8 per 100 people, while the US ranks first in the world with per capita gun ownership at 112.6 guns per 100 residents, as published in *The Telegraph* in October 2016.

The main difference is that Canada has stricter gun laws. In Canada, guns are classified into three categories, according to the Royal Canadian Mounted Police:

- Non-restricted: regular shotguns and rifles, and some military-style rifles and shotguns.

- Prohibited: most handguns that either have a short (less than 105 milimeters) barrel or are 32 or 25 caliber, full automatic weapons, guns with sawed-off barrels, and certain military rifles like the AK-47.

- Restricted: non-prohibited handguns, some semi-automatic rifles, and certain non-semi rifles as well.

All three kinds of guns can be purchased and owned legally (even "prohibited" ones), but the requirements for owning restricted and prohibited guns are much stricter.

GUN POLICIES IN CANADA

In Canada, every single gun owner must be licensed. The US does not have a federal license for gun owners. In Canada, you must register semi-automatics and hand guns with the government. Those applying for a license to own a non-restricted firearm must pass a series of firearms safety tests, and those applying for licensing covering restricted or prohibited firearms must pass another set of tests as well.

In Canada, a person must be 18 to get a license. However, minors aged 12 to 17 can possess non-restricted weapons if a licensed adult is responsible for them. In the US, there are states that actually prohibit gun registration and while some states have registration, the ones that don't have registration outnumber the ones that do.

Canadians applying for gun licenses "must pass background checks which consider criminal, mental, addiction and domestic violence records." In addition to criminal checks, this involves establishing that they had not been treated for a mental illness "associated with violence or threatened or attempted violence," or had a "history of behavior that includes violence or threatened or attempted violence on the part of the person against any person," within the past five years. Additionally, "third party character references for each gun license applicant are required," according to the Royal Canadian Mounted Police (RCMP, www.rcmp. grc.gc.ca).

Furthermore, Canada's background checks are done through one centralized database. In the US, the FBI gathers data from a number of sources and sometimes local mental health and criminal information. Additionally, a loophole in this process is that a criminal check must be done within three days and if it is not, then the applicant may obtain his firearm.

Canada forbids conceal carry and open carry unless these are part of the person's job. However, there is an exception to this. In very rare occasions, a person wishing to conceal-carry can be issued such a license for "protection of life," usually when there is a "an active police file and a verifiable threat, as well as police confirmation that they cannot provide adequate protection for that person."

To find out more about Canadian gun laws go to http://www.rcmp-grc.gc.ca/cfp-pcaf/index-eng.htm and http://www.rcmp-grc.gc.ca/cfp-pcaf/form-formulaire/index-eng.htm#f921. Please keep in mind that laws are subject to change.

What about Accidents with Guns?

Stricter gun laws, like those in Canada, could help reduce gun accidents. In Canada, guns must be kept locked and unloaded. Also, we can look at smart guns, which are programed only to be used by their owners. This would stop kids from getting shot by accident and would deter the stealing of guns.

Defending Ourselves without Guns

We can also defend ourselves without the use of guns, as there are many non-lethal and less lethal options that exist. These include pepper spray, tactical flashlights, stun guns, and Tasers. Bulletproof vests or items like bulletproof clip boards and back packs are other options. There is even a company that manufactures bulletproof clothing.

From a criminal justice standpoint, there is also technology called the "ammunition coding system." This assigns a unique code to every round of ammunition manufactured, and by recording sales records, law enforcement personnel are able to easily trace the ammunition involved in a crime and have a way to pursue and solve cases.

Study what other countries are doing to curb gun violence. A number of solutions already exist, but nothing will happen unless enough people get politically involved to elect those who want enact common-sense legislation.

In my opinion, the majority of U.S. citizens would welcome some form of greater regulation concerning guns. A breakdown of such regulations can be found in Chapter 19 of the book, *Reducing Gun Violence in America: Informing Policy with Evidence and Analysis*, published by the Center for Gun Policy and Research, Johns Hopkins University's Bloomberg School of Public Health, edited by Daniel W. Webster and Jon S. Varnick.

BULLETPROOF RESOURCES

Since not enough people have supported individuals running for public office who wish to enact common-sense gun laws, we are forced to look at alternative ways you can protect yourself from being shot. Please not that I have not personally tested any of the following products. Please also keep in mind that companies may come and go, so it's best if you conduct your own research into such resources.

According to Jason Hanson, former CIA operative and author of the book *Spy Secrets that Can Save Your Life,*

> Bulletproof panels can come in really handy and actually have a few uses. My bulletproof panel is level 3A,the same material that is used for the bulletproof vests worn by police officers. Level 3A is the highest level of protection you can get to protect yourself from blunt trauma and this is what you want in a high-risk situation.
>
> In the event there is an active shooter, I'm going to use the panel to protect my vital areas-and my life could be saved.

Another tool he recommends is QuickClot, which is basically gauze that's covered in a substance which accelerates the body's natural clotting process if one does get shot.

The Hardwire Whiteboard is a NIJ-level III bulletproof product. It is a dry-erase board with the capability of stopping a variety of handgun and shotgun projectiles. It comes in two sizes. The standard size can cover a person from head to toe when crouching. The large size can cover a person head to legs when crouching. Hardwire also produces a clipboard with NIJ III-level protection as well, which you can place in your briefcase, backpack, bag, or laptop case. Hardwire's website is www.hardwirellc.com .

Interceptor produces a deskpad that holds a IIIA bulletproof shield underneath the paper pad. It has a Dyneema/Spectra core. This allows it to decelerate and catch multiple hits from incoming bullets. They also produce a Home Defense Bulletproof IIA Shield with the same core as the desk pad. It has two nylon straps on its back along with an elastic band that can be used to run your arm through. Interceptor's website is www.bulletinterceptor.com

The Guard Dog ProShield II backpack uses lightweight IIIA armor and is designed for students, travelers, and professionals. It allows you to carry a laptop and portable electronics. It has plenty of organizational departments and an auxiliary audio cord connection that can route your music player's or phone's audio cable directly to a connection on its left shoulder strap to keep your audio wires from tangling. The company reports that the product has been tested against 9mm Luger and .44Magnum bullets. Its website is URL is www.guarddog-security.com.

Please note that I have not personally tested any of these products and that the field is growing constantly.

CHAPTER FOURTEEN

ELDER ABUSE / SELF-DEFENSE FOR SENIORS

The elderly can face many types of abuse. The abuse can include sexual abuse, physical abuse, psychological abuse, financial abuse, abandonment, and neglect. Below, we cover those abuses that impact the elderly physically and psychologically. Also, research shows that elders are more likely to be abused by their loved ones rather then by staff or paid workers, according to the Council on Aging.

PHYSICAL ABUSE OF THE ELDERLY

To completely know what physical abuse is we have to define it. It is the deliberate use of force against an elderly individual. The word *deliberate* is used because in some cases, legitimate restraint may include the use of force, like restraints, which then result in injury. The deliberate use of force may result in physical pain, injury, or impairment as a result of shoving, hitting, pushing, restraining, confining and an inappropriate use of drugs.

When determining elder abuse, one must distinguish between normal bruising patterns and those created by abuse. Normal or accidental bruises usually appear in a predictable fashion. They tend to be large and on the extremities. Some medications may also cause bruises to appear and in some cases, there will be multiple bruises and some bruises will look more severe.

Signs that can provide you with clues that abuse may exist include:

- Abused elders are likely to have bruises on head, neck or torso. Time is a factor when looking at bruising as they may change in color and appearance.

- Changes in the seniors' personality or behavior.

- Broken bones, sprains, welts, swelling, and dislocations.

- Wounds, cuts, abrasions, and burns.

- Unwarranted restraints, unexplained, or hidden injuries

- A caregiver's refusal for you to see the patient alone.

- The elder's clothing appears to be disheveled, soiled, torn or the person is not appropriately dressed for their environment.

- The elder has an appearance of being malnourished, hungry, confused, disoriented and/or has unexplained weight loss.

ELDER SEXUAL ABUSE

When sexual contact with an elderly person occurs without that person's consent, it is sexual elder abuse. Not only can this involve physical sex acts, but also the showing of pornographic materials, forcing the elderly to watch sex acts and or forcing the elderly to undress. If you feel that this might be the case, look for:

- Unexplained venereal disease or genital infection
- Bruises around genitals or breasts

♦ Bloody, torn, or stained undergarments

♦ Unexplained anal or vaginal bleeding

When someone you know is in this type of a situation, it is best to notify the authorities, like Adult Protective Services. If you are a family member, contact an experienced elder abuse attorney. Adult Protective Services also has a national presence. This is their link. http://www.napsa-now.org

Please keep in mind that you don't need a lot of evidence to report a case of elder abuse, but you should be as specific as possible.

Another national resource is The National Center on Elder Abuse (website www.ncea.aoa.gov), as well as the US Department of Health and Human Services. For further information on elder abuse, contact the National Committee for the Prevention of Elder Abuse (www.prevent-elderabuse.org). For cases that involve nursing homes, there is Nursing Home Abuse News. (www.elderly-abuse.com).

For those unable to access the Internet, the following are hotlines one can call.

♦ In the US: 1-800-677-1116
♦ In the UK: 08088088141
♦ In Ireland: 1-800-940-010
♦ In Australia: 1-300-651-192
♦ In South Africa: 080-111-2131

Please keep in mind that phone numbers are like websites and may change over time. When in doubt, contact your local elected official.

SELF-DEFENSE FOR SENIORS

The term "senior" can be very misleading. On the one hand, there is the definition imposed by society, usually around 55 and up. For our purposes, let's focus on mobility. A person can be 70-plus years old and still be mobile enough to effectively defend himself, or a 55-year-old couch potato who needs help walking. Either way, the same principles of self-defense apply:

1. Use your intuition.
2. Use verbal and psychological strategies.
3. If all else fails, use physical tactics to the best of your abilities..

As we age, our bodies limit what we can do physically. Therefore, the best self-defense in this stage of life is planning ahead. Select people you know and trust to look after you before you need assistance. Train them what to look for as signs of abuse, which could include bed sores, dehydration, and evidence of falling.

If you select a family member to look after you, make sure it will be that person and not someone else. Make sure you trust them. Sometimes it's the family that makes that decision because you are unable to. In some cases, that decision goes to a relative who will delegate it to their child, who is not interested in looking after the senior.

It is always good to select more than one person to be your confidant if you are in an assisted living facility or nursing home. Agree on a code word that you can use that means you need help. The word or words should be something simple but distinct like "my gold watch," the title of an old TV program, or even a passage from a favorite book. Develop a solid contact schedule. Agree to a specific time and place to meet at the location. Make sure you have access to a cell phone. This should not be a problem for the establishment unless you are suffering from a severe illness where it might be inappropriate.

Taking classes in Tai Chi Chuan, Chi Gong, or even ballroom dancing, can help maintain mobility and balance. According to the CDC, in 2016, falls were the leading cause of injury and death in older Americans. In China, a morning ritual is either doing Tai Chi or ballroom dancing. Some Tai Chi instructors are also versed in the martial art application of the Tai Chi moves. It is always good to keep active as long as one can.

Beware of individuals using tricks of distraction to get too close to you with the intent of robbing you. Have a drop wallet or drop purse to use and allow you to escape.

Age is not nor should be a restriction in learning self-defense. A number of Baby Boomers are active in the martial arts, as well as staying fit through a variety of activities, such as walking, swimming, or other sports.

For those who wish to focus more on developing their mind-body connection through Tai Chi or Chi Gong, do some research about instructors in your community.

It is always best to see what works well for you after you speak with your physician. Do activities that you enjoy and keep you healthy.

RESOURCES AND REFERENCES

Being Safe: Using Psychological and Emotional Readiness to Avoid Being a Victim of Violence and Crime by Edward M. Ross

Fear Less: Real Truth About Risk, Safety, and Security in a Time of Terrorism by Gavin de Becker

How to Protect yourself from Crime by Ira Lipman

Humane Pressure Point Self-Defense: Dillman Pressure Point Method for Law Enforcement, Medical Personnel, Business Professionals, Men and Women by George A. Dillman and Chris Thomas

Protecting the Gift: Keeping Children and Teenagers Safe (and Parents Sane) by Gavin de Becker

Reducing Gun Violence in America: Informing Policy with Evidence and Analysis, edited by Daniel W. Webster and Jon S. Vernick

Risk Factors for Femicide in Abusive Relationships: Results From a Multisite Case Control Study by Jacquline Campbell, et al. See. https://www.ncbi.nlm.nih.gov/pmc/articles/PMC1447915/

Scaling Force: Dynamic Decision Making Under Threat of Violence by Rory Miller and Lawrence A. Kane

So I Won't Have to Fight: Bully Solutions from Martial Arts Masters by Brad Scornsvscco

Spy Secrets That Can Save Your Life: A Former CIA Officer Reveals Safety and Survival Techniques to Keep You and Your Family Protected by Jason Hanson

Strong on Defense by Sanford Strong

The Gift of Fear and Other Survival Signals that Protect Us from Violence by Gavin de Becker

The Last Gun: How Changes in the Gun Industry are Killing Americans and What It Will Take to Stop It by Tom Diaz

The Second Amendment: A Biography by Michael Waldman

Acknowledgments

I would like to offer special thanks to those who have set me on my path: Bruce Lee, Vladimir Vasiliev, and Chris Thomas.

In addition, I would like to thank HenschelHaus for accepting this work and to Kira Henschel for her steadfast dedication to the project.

ABOUT THE AUTHOR

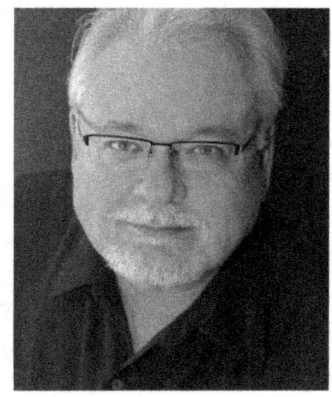

Wes Manko is one of America's foremost experts in self-defense and violence prevention. He is the owner and chief instructor of DEFENSE-WORKS, a company specializing in conducting violence prevention, personal safety, and self-defense workshops to non-profits organizations,, businesses, law enforcement, military, civilians, and individuals.

He began studying martial arts over thirty years ago. His journey has led him to obtain experience in police defensive tactics, aikido, tae kwon do, fencing, boxing, chin na, tai chi chuan, aiki-jitsu, Chinese kempo, ryukyu kempo, kyusho jitsu, combat hapkido, and Systema Russian martial art.

He has been certified to teach Systema Russian Martial Art by Vladimir Vasiliev, the co-founder, director, and chief instructor for Systema and a ten-year veteran of the special operations unit of the SPETSNAZ (Russian special forces).

Wes combines this knowledge with an academic background that includes an Associate Degree in Police Science, a Bachelor's Degree in Criminal Justice, and a Master's Degree in Public Administration to produce a solid, reality-based approach to speaking and training in self-defense. In other words, he only teaches the stuff that works.

Additionally, Mr. Manko has been published nationally in *Black Belt* magazine, *Self-Defense for Women* magazine, and @LAW, a publication for legal professionals.

On November 9, 2005, Mr. Manko was awarded a citation from the Assembly of the State of Wisconsin for providing a wide array of courses that have aided law enforcement, military, and civilian personnel, including victims of domestic violence and sexual abuse, as well as his outstanding service to the community through providing lifesaving instruction in violence prevention and realistic self-defense training.

To schedule a workshop or purchase additional products,
Mr. Manko can be reached
through his website : www.defenseworks.us or
email at wes@defenseworks.us.

CPSIA information can be obtained
at www.ICGtesting.com
Printed in the USA
FSHW04n1047070318
45215FS